GW00375237

THE POW
POSITIVE EATING

ABOUT THE AUTHORS

Amanda Wynne
MSc, BSc (Hons), PG Dip Diet, RD

Amanda is a registered dietitian from the UK; she has university qualifications in catering and applied nutrition; in dietetics; and in health sciences. Amanda has had extensive experience in working for the food industry, both in the UK and in New Zealand and she has also been an advocate for the dietetic profession on both sides of the world. Amanda developed an interest in weight loss when she edited the *British Nutrition Foundation Task Force Report on Obesity*, and since then she has co-authored *The Nutrition Handbook for Community Nurses* and has written numerous articles on many aspects of food and nutrition. Amanda makes regular appearances on TV and on the radio to promote food and nutrition.

Alison Crawshaw
DipPhty, ManipPhys, MNZSP

Alison is a registered physiotherapist from New Zealand. Having followed countless diets since her weight problems began at the age of 13, Alison has many years' experience of the weight management strategies that do and don't work. She also has a deep understanding of the emotional and psychological issues that go hand in hand with being overweight. As a qualified physiotherapist she believes that, along with a healthy diet, exercise plays a vital part in maintaining weight loss.

THE WEBSITE

www.thepowerofpositiveeating.com is the website the authors have set up for the readers of this book. Any queries or comments about the website should be directed to Alison Crawshaw via the website and not via the publishers of this book.

THE POWER OF

POSITIVE EATING

HOW TO LOSE WEIGHT AND ENJOY A HEALTHY LIFE

Amanda Wynne and
Alison Crawshaw

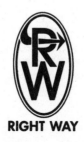

RIGHT WAY

Copyright notice

© 2004 Amanda Wynne and Alison Crawshaw.
The authors assert their moral rights in the work.
First published in New Zealand by Reed Books, a division of Reed
Publishing (NZ) Ltd., 2002.

All rights reserved. No part of this book may be reproduced, stored
in a retrieval system, or transmitted, in any form or by any means,
electronic, photocopying, mechanical, recording or otherwise, without the prior permission of the copyright owner.

Conditions of sale
This book shall only be sold, lent, or hired, for profit, trade, or
otherwise, in its original binding, except where special permission
has been granted by the Publisher.

Whilst care is taken in selecting Authors who are authoritative in
their subjects, it is emphasised that their books can reflect their
knowledge only up to the time of writing. Information can be
superseded and printers' errors can creep in. This book is sold,
therefore, on the condition that neither Publisher nor Author can be
held legally responsible for the consequences of any error or
omission there may be.

Typeset in 11/12 pt Times New Roman by Letterpart Ltd., Reigate,
Surrey. Printed and bound in Great Britain by Cox & Wyman Ltd.,
Reading, Berkshire.

The *Right Way* series is published by Elliot Right Way Books,
Brighton Road, Lower Kingswood, Tadworth, Surrey, KT20 6TD,
U.K. For information about our company and the other books we
publish, please visit our website at www.right-way.co.uk

CONTENTS

INTRODUCTION

Give a man a fish and he will eat for a day.
Teach a man to fish and he will eat for the rest of his life.

CHINESE PROVERB

You'll have noticed that many diet books consist largely of precise lists of foods and meals that you are expected to eat in order to lose weight. While following such a prescription for weight loss will almost certainly work in the short term, as soon as you come off the diet your weight will go back on again. Why? There are several reasons: you're not learning new eating habits; you're not necessarily eating the foods that you like; you're following a plan based on someone else's food preferences; and, perhaps most importantly, you're not addressing the underlying reasons for your overeating.

So what do we mean by the power of positive eating? After reading this book, you will digest the information and strategies that underpin a new lifestyle with a positive attitude to food and the ability to manage your weight for the rest of your life. The principle behind the book is a variation on the Chinese proverb above; we would say: *Give someone a meal plan and he or she will lose weight for a week. Teach someone new eating and lifestyle habits, and the weight loss will last a lifetime.*

The power of positive eating strategy offers more than a set of meal plans or a restricted list of foods. It is a holistic approach to eating and weight control, that has been jointly written by a qualified dietitian and a successful dieter.

The latest information on dieting and food choices is presented along with some frank discussion of dieting and being overweight. We look at why we eat, the psychological and social issues, and set out techniques to lose weight and keep it off for the rest of your life.

This book takes just a few hours of your life to read and absorb, yet will give you back years in return as you develop a positive attitude, lose that excess weight and experience the health benefits. It will empower you – mind, body and soul – to move forward from where you are now.

To our knowledge, this is the first time a book has been jointly written by a dietitian and someone actually on a weight loss programme. The combination of accurate scientific information and personal insights is therefore unique to this book. We know the power of positive eating philosophy will inspire you, motivate you, and help you succeed where you have failed in the past.

During the development of the power of positive eating strategy, several people tried out the programme. Here are some of their comments:

'People keep commenting on how phenomenal I look and ask how I did it. I tell them it was easy and that I have only had to make a few changes and adaptations to my life to fit in the exercise and modify what I eat.'

'It's not about deprivation – it's about gaining a life! Every diet I have been on in the past involved me feeling like my throat had been cut, and I felt hard done by because I wasn't eating what I wanted. What I have learnt from the power of positive eating is that you can have a life, and eat well. Not once have I felt I am "on a diet".'

'My doctor was amazed, I am now so much healthier. I had high blood pressure and was on the verge of having to go on medication, but thanks to the weight loss my blood pressure is now normal.'

'The power of positive eating has opened my eyes and I'm moving forward. It has given me the 'know how' and the motivation to change my eating habits and my thoughts. Now I can really say I am coping and that success is on the way! My eyes are now open, the weight is moving and I am smiling!'

'I've lost 10 kilos in 10 weeks, this is no diet! I can now play actively with my children and I have so much more energy.'

'The book is a great help, and the recipes are fantastic. I exercise three times a week now, by brisk walking for 45 minutes at a time. I would recommend the book to everyone, but it must be said that willpower plays a big part in any diet/exercise regime.'

'I have found the power of positive eating strategy to be immensely helpful in planning my eating and food intake. I run a very busy and successful company and don't have much time to spend in the kitchen preparing meals. The practical recipe and meal planning ideas have helped me to eat healthily in a way that is quick and easy.'

'It's all about a new attitude and way of life – this whole strategy fits in really well with my busy lifestyle. I found it easy to shed a few pounds, and to keep trim and fit with the information in the book and on the website.'

'Recently, I woke up to the threat of heart disease, diabetes, and dying well before my time! I'm delighted to say that I've lost 8 kilos in the first 8 weeks of following the power of positive eating plan. I was 207 kilos and now I'm 199 kilos; I feel as though I have made a great start and that the changes have been relatively easy to implement.'

'I have found that the power of positive eating has really helped me to lose weight; so far I have lost 5 kilos which is great. I have changed my eating habits quite significantly, making small gradual changes that I can keep to, and I am more attentive to what I eat in general.'

1

THE POWER OF POSITIVE EATING PHILOSOPHY

Congratulations! By starting to read this book you've taken the very first steps to a whole new life. Now read on and learn just what the power of positive eating is about.

When looking at a lifelong solution to weight control, simply telling you all about healthy eating probably won't do you much good. Everyone knows by now that cream cakes are full of fat and calories, and that fruit and vegetables are good for you! The power of positive eating is not a prescriptive diet, but is a whole new approach that gets to the root of the problem and provides real solutions. All that's required of you is that you spend a few hours of your life reading this book. You will then have the information you need to manage your weight for the rest of your life. The aim of the power of positive eating is *permanent* weight loss. You can achieve this – you just need to acquire the knowledge to do it, and then put it into action.

YOU'RE NOT ALONE

A lot of people who successfully lose weight and maintain that weight loss manage to do so as they have a good network of support. Look to your family and friends for support, and look to develop new interests and activities. You could also log on to our website at www.thepowerof positiveeating.com for help, ideas and information.

UNDERSTANDING WHAT'S GOING ON

On the face of it, the solution to being overweight seems simple. If you consume more energy (calories) than you burn up, you will put on weight. Conversely, if you burn up more energy than you consume, you will lose weight. Unsympathetic friends or relatives often tell us to 'just go on a diet' if we need to lose weight. This shows they don't realise how hard it really is. Many people don't understand that there's a great deal more to lasting weight loss than just dieting.

We need to grasp not only the effects of different foods and nutrients, but also the complex biological, social and psychological issues involved. If it really was that simple to lose those unwanted pounds, then far fewer people would have a weight problem in the first place. Unravelling and understanding the different aspects of weight control is an essential first step to achieving lifelong success.

WHAT'S THE MENU FOR THE POWER OF POSITIVE EATING?

The power of positive eating is based on the latest information, with complex jargon simplified into language that everyone can understand.

There are four key reasons why the power of positive eating plan will help you succeed:

1. It identifies and addresses the reasons you are eating too much, rather than just telling you what to eat.

2. It offers an understanding of basic nutrition and food principles so that you can adapt the foods you like to eat to a healthy, lower calorie-eating pattern.

3. It helps you find easy and enjoyable ways to get active and burn off that extra weight.

4. It suggests how to gain help and support from those around you, and gives you the chance to make new friends.

To start with, we look at how to tell if you are truly overweight. You'll find out how to measure and monitor your weight, and some of the barriers and difficulties associated with losing weight. Then we look at the health factors. While we do need to become more accepting of our bodies, and to promote acceptance among others, we also need to appreciate the health risks of being severely overweight. A healthier, happier life is certainly a good motivating factor in the struggle to lose weight.

Many of us turn to food when we feel unhappy or stressed, because we find comfort in eating. But the truth is, if we can take the focus in our lives away from food, we can find fulfilment in many other interests and activities. We look at what motivates us to overeat, and ways of addressing this.

We'll also address the triggers to eating, such as habit and boredom, and addictions to foods like chocolate. It is important to understand how to cope with these. Dieting should not be about consuming an endless round of cottage cheese and limp lettuce – you will initially lose weight this way, but it's not sustainable in the long term. Eating is an experience that should be enjoyed and relished. What's wrong with chips, ice cream and choco-lates? They are fine as the occasional treat, and if the diet is to be followed on a lifelong basis, rather than just temporarily, then of course these foods can be included in limited amounts if you enjoy them. The most impor-tant message is to get the balance of the overall diet right and to consume appropriate portion sizes and quantities of the right sorts of foods.

The real key, though, is to change your behaviour. This is challenging, especially after many years of following a particular pattern. However, we set out strategies to help you move on from old habits and routines.

We'll then focus on the nitty-gritty of food and what happens when you eat. There are many short-term diets that follow the same tired old formula, claiming to have found *the* system that will help achieve that permanent and previously elusive weight loss. Others offer miracle cures, in which we will magically slim down just by eating foods in particular combinations, or by omitting particular foods. Nice ideas, and a real shame they're a load of rubbish! It's true that many of these set patterns do help you lose weight for a limited period, but only because you are eating fewer calories, not because of any magical combination of foods. Unfortunately, the weight nearly always piles back on once the diet is over, and you often put on more weight than you've lost. You've probably tried many of these diets yourself so far. We'll give you the expert low-down on different diets and the reasons why they do or don't work. This should help you understand your past dieting disasters and successes.

We outline a balanced diet and the food-group approach to healthy eating. You'll be pleased to hear that calorie-counting is no longer necessary. By becoming familiar with nutrients, food groups, portion sizes and meal plans you will be able to eat the right type of foods, not just now but long into the future. With this approach you won't isolate yourself by having to prepare and eat a funny combination of foods while your family eats normally. Your whole family will benefit from these new and enjoyable eating patterns (although young children and those with special dietary requirements do need to be considered separately).

There is plenty of practical advice on every aspect of your new approach to eating, from food-shopping and nutrition labels, to cooking equipment, meal plans and portion sizes, and we provide lots of delicious, healthy recipe ideas for you and your family. We also counter common food myths with the cold hard facts.

Then we tackle that other really important issue: exercise! Exercise is one of the key factors in losing weight and maintaining that loss, because it helps burn up the calories. It also brings numerous health benefits, and can be an enjoyable way to spend time with others, or on your own.

We are far less active today than in previous generations,

and we don't need to read the scientific studies to know there is a strong relationship between inactivity and weight problems. But just as an example, it's been shown that people who watch more television are more likely to have weight problems. You may have preconceived ideas about exercise, and envision yourself struggling in a trendy aerobics studio full of super-fit gym-junkies with perfect bodies. This is an understandable concern, but gyms today are full of people of all shapes, sizes and fitness levels. Even if you still feel reluctant, there are lots of other places to get fit. Exercise is for everyone, and we suggest ways of getting more activity into your life in a gradual and enjoyable way.

Many of us lead busy, stressful lives, which leave little time for ourselves. To help you relax and get in touch with your spiritual side we set out some breathing and relaxation techniques. It's vital that you feel good about your inner self if you are fully to enjoy a life free of worry about food.

The prevailing attitudes towards obesity have been described as the last remaining socially acceptable form of prejudice.[1] We discuss the importance of supporting those friends who are aiming to lose weight, and of working together to try and encourage a change in people's perceptions.

Finally, we summarise all the key points you need to remember, with advice on putting it all together. You will be able to dip into Chapter 13 over the coming months to remind yourself of your new direction in life.

WHAT YOU WILL ACHIEVE
When you have digested the power of positive eating philosophy you will:

❖ Be able to implement a new way of eating and living with a positive attitude towards food.

❖ Have a good level of knowledge on the different fad diets and miracle cures and understand what does and doesn't work.

❖　Be ready to start an action plan that is fun and will help burn off those extra calories, resulting in weight loss.

❖　Have an insight into psychological factors and what motivates us to change.

❖　Have the confidence to seek support from family and/or friends.

❖　Have the knowledge, tools and understanding to lose weight and maintain that weight loss for the rest of your life, with a whole new enjoyable, revitalised and active lifestyle.

2

A TIME BOMB: HEALTH RISKS

Many of us who have a bit of weight to lose feel isolated and alone, surrounded by magazines, movies and television shows featuring women with stick-like figures. But despite these media images, the obesity rate has more than doubled in many countries over the last 20 years, and it has been estimated by the International Obesity Task Force that around 300 million people in the world today are clinically obese.[1]

In countries such as the USA and the UK, at least one in every two people needs to lose some weight. You may be shocked and alarmed by the latest statistics on the increasing number of people who are having difficulties with their weight. You'll also be reassured that you're not the only one with a problem.

One reason the number of overweight people has increased in the developed world is that while our environment has changed dramatically since the Stone Age, our bodies have not evolved at the same rate. To get enough food for survival, our ancestors had to go hunting or gathering, which required a lot of energy: that's what our bodies are geared up for. We are designed to survive under conditions where food is scarce. However, where there is an abundance of food and no pressing need to take any exercise, these biological mechanisms have no use, and it's very easy to put on more weight than we need.

We certainly need to tackle the problem now before it's too late. The growing threat to our health is like a time bomb ticking away.

It's interesting to note that during the same period of increasing obesity, there has been an explosion in the diet industry. Almost every week some new diet or miracle cure is promoted in magazines, newspapers, bookshops and on television. However, this doesn't mean that fewer of us are overweight – in fact, as we know, the opposite is true. As the number of diets has increased, so has the number of overweight people. You may think there's something a little odd about this, and you'd be right.

The fact is: short-term dieting makes you fat. You can lose weight on a slimming diet, but it takes a great deal of stamina and hard work. Then when you finish the diet or give up on it, and return to your normal eating habits, the weight piles back on. Unfortunately you acquire a little more weight each time, so your weight is actually going *up* through dieting, not down! One recent study found that fewer than one in 20 people managed to lose weight and keep it off over a three-year period.[2]

Constantly trying different diets isn't good for you. To keep your weight down in the long term requires a different approach, but let's begin by seeing how overweight you really are and what the risks are for your health.

OVERWEIGHT OR OBESE?

To most people, obesity is just another word for being fat, which has very negative overtones. To health professionals, however, there's a big difference between being overweight and being 'clinically obese'. If you are clinically obese you face big health risks. Being overweight is less risky, but you could tip over into that obese category if you are not careful.

How do you tell if you are clinically obese, or just overweight? Here are two ways to assess your weight, and what this means for you.

Body Mass Index

This is a useful method commonly used by health professionals. It was first developed by a Belgian astronomer called Quetelet, who noticed that in adults of normal build, weight was proportional to height; in other words, the taller you are, the more you weigh. Once the figure, or index, is calculated, it's translated into the level of risk to your health. This is a useful measurement for men and women of all ages, but it does have some drawbacks. Those who are very muscular, body builders for example, may have a high index without an increased risk to health. For most of us though, this is certainly a useful indication of health risk. To avoid complex calculations, follow the steps below.

1. WEIGH YOURSELF without shoes and wearing light indoor clothing. You will need an accurate set of scales to measure your weight. If you don't have one, visit your local pharmacy, gym or health centre.

2. MEASURE YOUR HEIGHT.

3. Using the chart overleaf, LINE UP YOUR HEIGHT AND WEIGHT MEASUREMENTS. This will show whether you are underweight, OK, overweight, fat or very fat.

4. Now have a LOOK AT THE PANEL on page 21 showing what this means for your health.

Are you overweight?

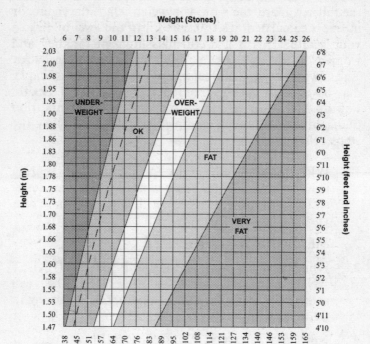

Reproduced by the kind permission of the Food Standards Agency, UK.

Body Mass Index and Your Health

UNDERWEIGHT: You may need advice from a dietitian on how to increase your weight to a healthy level. Aim for a good balanced diet based on the principles outlined in this book, and increase your food intake.

OK: You are the ideal weight for your height, and should not face any health risks. However, if your weight is to the left of the dotted line, you may be at risk of becoming underweight. Aim to have a healthy balanced diet and make sure you don't lose any more weight.

OVERWEIGHT: At this level there is a slightly increased risk to health. If you are towards the upper end of the range you may wish to consider losing weight, as there is a risk you may tip over into the obese category. The guidelines set out in this book will help you to trim down a little.

FAT: You are classed as clinically obese. You may tire easily, and become short of breath. This is because of the excess weight you're carrying around. You are also at increased risk from the diseases listed later in this chapter. You should seriously consider losing weight.

VERY FAT: You are classed as morbidly obese. There is a very significant risk of the diseases listed later in this chapter, and you may already be suffering from a number of these. You are likely to be severely restricted in performing normal activities and your life expectancy is reduced. You would benefit enormously from losing weight. The information in this book will certainly help you, and increase your understanding of the issues involved. You may also find it useful to seek specialised advice from a registered dietitian.

Waist Measurement
Recent scientific evidence has suggested that simply measuring the size of your waist can be enough to tell you if your weight poses a risk to your health. Using a standard tape measure, stand up and measure round your waist where your belt would normally go. Now check the figures in the chart below to find out your health status.

Waist Measurement and Health Risk		
MEN	*Increased risk*	94cm (37 inches) or more
	Substantial risk	102cm (40 inches) or more
WOMEN	*Increased risk*	80cm (32 inches) or more
	Substantial risk	88cm (35 inches) or more

MEASURING OBESITY IN CHILDREN
Body mass index and waist measurements are suitable only for adults. For children, special growth charts are used. If you're concerned about your child's weight you should consult your doctor. You may be referred to a registered dietitian for specialist advice. It is important to pay careful attention to the diets of overweight and obese children, as excess restriction of food intake could reduce intake of nutrients too much and impair growth and development.

A FRUITY APPROACH
The way we store our fat results in two main body shapes, as shown opposite. They are sometimes referred to as the apple shape, where fat is stored in the tummy area, and the pear shape, where it is stored in the hips and thighs.

Men and postmenopausal women are more often apple shaped, and younger women pear shaped, although this is not always the case. You need to know which shape you are, as the health risks vary. Being apple shaped carries more health risks. The good news for 'apples' though, is that they seem to lose weight more easily.

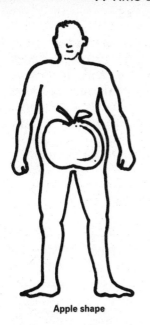

Apple shape

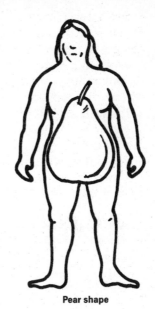

Pear shape

A BEAUTIFUL BODY

What motivates most of us to lose weight is to look good; we want to be admired by our friends and desired by our lovers. We live in a society that sees slimness as a sign of beauty and success. Many of us aspire to a slender figure similar to that of the supermodels, whose heavenly bodies adorn all the glossy magazines. You need to realise, though, that only a tiny proportion of the population can ever actually look like that. In actual fact, your body shape is largely down to your genes. Typically, women have a pear-shaped figure, storing weight in our lower half, and to aim to look like a supermodel is an unrealistic goal. But we can aim to look our best, and to achieve a trim figure by having a good diet and a healthy lifestyle.

WOMEN'S PROBLEMS ...

It's not just overweight women who think they are too fat; just about all women worry about their weight. This was demonstrated in an interesting paper in *Nutrition Today*,[3] which reported on a *Glamour* magazine reader survey carried out some years ago. The survey looked at how 33,000 women felt about their bodies, and the results showed that three out of four felt too fat. In fact, only one in four were actually overweight, and a significant number were underweight. This distorted perception of our own bodies is a real concern, and there is no sign today, in the twenty-first century, that our self-esteem is improving.

Of course we need to feel good about ourselves and be at a weight that feels comfortable. However, unnecessary dieting and obsession with weight can be harmful.

... AND MEN'S

Fat is a feminist issue – so goes the famous saying by psychotherapist Susie Orbach.[4] This may well be true, but it totally ignores the effect of unrealistic body images on poor old men! Traditionally men have been the onlookers in this whole sorry 'weight-obsession' affair, but times are certainly changing, and men are increasingly being targeted themselves. After much criticism of her figure, in 1998 Barbie developed a thicker waist, more proportional hips and a smaller mouth and bust, but action toys for boys are getting more muscular as time goes by.[5] To add to this, a barrage of men's magazines has appeared in recent years, exploiting men's insecurities with their 'fat-fighting, muscle-building, six-pack stomach' ideals. While there is an increasing awareness of the damaging effects of an unrealistic body image on girls, the feelings that boys might have are often forgotten. Men do need help too, because although they may seem just to take it on the chin, deep down they can feel just the same way about their fat bodies as women.

AN UNHEALTHY STATE OF AFFAIRS

For many younger people, being affected by obesity-related illnesses often seems like a lifetime away. Usually it isn't until we hit our forties that health suddenly becomes an issue. It's at about this age that you might really start to notice things like tiredness, breathlessness, back pain, arthritis, sweatiness, and poor sleeping, as well as depression and period problems. As the following list shows, there are a number of quite serious health problems that are linked to being obese.

The fact is obesity can kill. Perhaps not directly, but certainly by increasing significantly the risk of potentially fatal illnesses such as heart disease, stroke and cancer. It has been estimated by the International Obesity Task Force that a severely obese person aged 25 to 35 is 12 times more likely to die than a slim person.[6] Further, a weight loss of 0.5–9kg (1–20 lb) in overweight women has been found to reduce deaths from obesity-related cancers by up to half, and diabetes-related deaths by around a third, in a 12-year study in the USA. Even reducing your weight a little can have great benefits.

Major Health Risks Associated With Obesity

❖ Adult-onset diabetes	❖ Breathing problems
❖ Heart disease	❖ Varicose veins
❖ Stroke	❖ Hernias
❖ High blood pressure	❖ Dermatitis
❖ High cholesterol	❖ Sleep problems
❖ Cancer	❖ Reproductive problems
❖ Back pain	❖ Pregnancy complications
❖ Arthritis	❖ Surgery complications
❖ Gout	❖ Depression

Diabetes

Diabetes is a disease where the body cannot produce enough insulin, the hormone that controls sugar levels in the blood. There are two types: juvenile-onset and adult-onset.

The risk of developing adult-onset diabetes in middle-aged people who are well into the clinically obese category can be as much as 100 times greater in women and 40 times greater in men than for a slim person. It has been estimated that 85–95 per cent of adult-onset diabetes is directly related to excess body fat.[7] The unlucky people who develop diabetes must pay very careful attention to diet and lifestyle, and may need medication or injections of insulin every day. If you can manage to lose weight, the likelihood that you will go on to develop diabetes is greatly reduced.

Heart Disease and Stroke
The risks of heart disease and stroke are greater in obese people. This is because when you have a lot of extra body fat you tend to have higher cholesterol levels and blood pressure. Weight loss can help reduce these.

Cancer
Obese people are at higher risk of certain types of cancer. Particularly in women who are postmenopausal, the risk of breast cancer is increased. The incidence of cancer of the womb, ovaries, cervix and gall bladder is also higher. In obese men, there is a greater risk of cancer of the colon, rectum and prostate.

Reproductive Problems
In obese girls, periods often start early, and period problems are more common. Obesity is also a major cause of infertility. Weight loss can help maintain normal periods and regulate ovulation. Women who are overweight should try to slim down before getting pregnant; otherwise if they cut down on foods too much during the pregnancy they may end up with a poor nutritional status. Obese pregnant women are at increased risk of diabetes during the pregnancy, and often have high blood pressure. Difficulties in giving birth are also more common among this group.

Other Health Problems

Modest levels of weight loss (about 5–10kg, or 11–22 lb) can improve lung function by reducing breathlessness, reduce joint and back pains, and aid proper sleep.[8]

We need to become more accepting of our bodies, with a realistic self-image and sensible eating patterns. However, if you are obese, there is a very real risk to your health, and it is important to reduce your weight. This is not simple: if it were, there would not be such a massive number of people battling their weight. In the last few years it has become obvious that short-term dieting is not the solution. Most people who struggle to lose weight already know a great deal about foods and dieting. What is perhaps less well known is the complex interaction between the factors that lead to weight gain. Weight loss is tricky, and carefully planned solutions are needed. These are explained in the next chapters.

3

HAPPINESS ON A PLATE?

While you may begin a diet successfully, with most of the tried and tested approaches it's only a matter of time before you simply run out of steam! There are lots of reasons why this may happen, but basically it's because managing your weight isn't about food at all, it's more about how you feel.

The truth is, although you may think you can find happiness on a plate, and that food can solve your problems – whether it's work stress, anxiety or a feeling of being unloved – you need to explore other ways to fulfil your needs.

As we all know, once you've decided to diet you become totally focused on food. Feeling perpetually hungry, you'll find yourself savouring every meal and snack, and spending inordinate amounts of time thinking of the next opportunity to eat. This is just human nature, but you need to shift your thoughts and energy to other areas (for more on different choices, read on, and see Chapter 11).

REASONS FOR EATING

Have you ever thought seriously about the situations that trigger your need to eat? Often, one of the least common reasons for eating is actual hunger. Educating yourself to eat primarily when you're hungry can help in the control of your weight. Learn to recognise hunger – that growly, empty feeling in your stomach – rather than following other cues. Realise there is a difference between being 'hungry' and being 'foody', that is wanting food for reasons other than hunger.

Palatability

Do you often eat simply because the food looks and tastes good? If you weren't hungry and were offered a bowl of raw vegetables, would you decline? What about if you were offered a bowl of chocolates – could you resist? Think about whether your eating is driven by internal signals, such as hunger, or external signals such as the palatability of food. If you can educate yourself to eat only when you're hungry, this can help in the control of your weight.

Addicted to Food

Some people claim to be addicted to certain foods; this is particularly common for women who are premenstrual or pregnant.

In the 1970s the idea was proposed that people crave carbohydrate foods such as bread and potatoes because carbohydrate raises the levels of serotonin, a chemical that can reduce feelings of depression. Although some experimental studies have shown some positive effects from carbohydrates, for those of us consuming a normal diet there is no clear evidence of any benefit. Beware of diets that claim a 'mood-lifting' effect from eating these foods.

Chocolate is perhaps the food most commonly claimed to be addictive. Studies have looked at the magnesium content, the caffeine, and the effect of stimulating endorphins (feel-good chemicals) in the body. However, overall it is thought that the craving for chocolate is a sensory one, rather than being linked to any one ingredient.[1] In other words, it seems that we eat it because it looks, tastes and smells great, although it would be interesting to see more research into this area.

The most likely cause of an addiction to food is the delicious taste of high-sugar, high-fat foods. The strategy for dealing with food cravings should be to try and find substitute foods to eat instead. Here are some suggestions:

❖ Chocolate cravings: have a low-calorie hot chocolate drink made with skimmed milk instead, or the occasional small portion of low-fat chocolate ice cream.

❖ Sweet cravings: have sugar-free chewing gum instead.

❖ Potato chip cravings: have popcorn instead.

❖ Cheese cravings: try the low-fat varieties instead. Buy much smaller quantities, grate and sprinkle it over food as flavouring rather than serving large amounts.

Eating to Feel Good
It is now well recognised that eating is closely linked to our emotions. We experience this as newborns, when our mother is our source of milk and love, and right through childhood, where sweets, chocolates and our favourite foods are given as rewards, to comfort us, as a token of love and affection. It's no wonder then that we turn to such foods for emotional reasons as adults when there are gaps in our lives – job dissatisfaction, lack of a partner, a feeling of vulnerability. Once we can recognise the emotional triggers in our own lives for seeking solace in food, we can look at changing our old habits.

Emotional Reasons for Eating	
❖ Depressed	❖ Vulnerable
❖ Upset	❖ Bored
❖ Anxious	❖ Needing instant gratification
❖ Angry	❖ Feeling unloved
❖ Stressed out	❖ Celebration
❖ Happy	❖ As a reward
❖ Lonely	

KEEPING TRACK OF FOOD AND FEELINGS
To understand the cues to eating, why not keep a diary? Buy a pocket notebook and write down when you eat,

what you eat and how you're feeling at the time, as shown in the following example:

Food	Amount	Time	Feelings
Chocolate bar	150g bar	Morning tea	Anxious
Scone	1	Late-morning snack	Bored
Ham salad sandwich	1 round	Lunch	Hungry
Sweets	Bumper pack	Throughout the day	Didn't think
Crisps	4 packs	Lunch, mid-afternoon, evening	Bored
Chocolate biscuits	3	Lunch	Lonely

For this to work you need to be honest with yourself: write down everything, it all counts. Stick to your normal habits, so you can figure out where you're at; don't change what you are eating just because you are writing it down. Record things as you go, rather than relying on memory. Be specific about what you have eaten and how you're feeling. Once you have a good record of your own reasons for eating, you can begin to address the issues in your life, as discussed below.

Boredom

Have you noticed that the urge to eat is exacerbated if you're bored? The need for a distraction at work often leads to snacking, popping out to the bakery for a cake, or worse, dipping into the biscuit tin whether you are hungry or not, often without even realising it. The same can be true if you're bored at home, and have a pantry stocked with delicious treats.

Learn to recognise this and do something about it. At work, you could talk to your manager to see if there are courses or training you can get involved with to make your job more exciting. Can you be given more responsibility? If this isn't possible it might be worth looking for a new job that makes more use of your talents and abilities. There's nothing like being busy to take the focus off food.

At home, look for things to occupy you so that you can't eat at the same time: having a long soak in the bath, gardening, calling your friends, or even working out with an exercise video.

Low Self-esteem
In a society that despises fatness and promotes a waif-like image as the ideal, we are constantly made to feel ashamed of our bodies if they don't conform to this perfection. This is probably why so many of us are on perpetual diets, whether we need to lose weight or not!

Working on how we see ourselves is actually very important in improving our self-esteem. We need to learn self-acceptance, despite having a physique that might not be like the ideal. Rather than poring over glossy fashion magazines, look around you at other normal people on the street, or at high-profile figures such as politicians and business leaders.

Also, you need to move away from that concept, 'If only I could lose a stone, I'd be happy', and set realistic goals: a size 10 might just not be attainable for your body shape; after all, we all have different-sized frames and different heights. And don't forget, all these celebrities and supermodels have thousands of dollars to spend on personal trainers, beauticians, plastic surgeons and of course expensive photographers who use the latest computer technology to touch up their imperfections on any publicity shots.

Focus on the positives. Of course we all have aspects of our appearance that we don't like, but we also have many good features, whether it's beautiful eyes, perfect nails or great legs. Learn to pay attention to these, and take the focus off your perceived flaws. Think about your non-physical attributes too. Maybe you have a great sense of humour and the ability to make people laugh; maybe you have great empathy and can help people solve their problems or achieve their aspirations; maybe you are musical, or an excellent cook, or are skilled at crafts. Recognising your own talents and abilities will help raise your self-esteem.

Get together with other people who wish to lose weight. Support from our peers is a great way to gain self-acceptance and improve self-esteem. With the help of others you can:

❖ Find the right shops to buy clothes that actually fit, and go on group shopping expeditions.

❖ Share skills in dressmaking.

❖ Get involved in group activities such as walking, dancing, cycling or even going to the gym.

❖ Visit the local beauty salon for ego-boosting beauty treats such as manicures, pedicures, facials and make-overs.

❖ Help each other with make-up and clothes tips.

We all come in different shapes and sizes and we really need to work together to gain acceptance of ourselves and of others.

Feeling Unloved
Following an argument with your partner, or after being dumped for someone several years younger or several pounds lighter, or simply because you're feeling lonely or vulnerable, it's common enough to retreat to bed with a large bowl of chocolate fudge ice cream or some other indulgent delight, seeking solace in food.

A lack of love and affection can often lead us to food, and this isn't surprising. Fancy meals are often a part of courtship – on Valentine's Day traditionally we give chocolate as a sign of our love, and some foods such as oysters and kiwi fruit are even suggested to be aphrodisiacs. Besides, food is always there should we need it, available and reliable. While there's nothing wrong with indulging now and again, if eating becomes a compensation for every little relationship problem, it can lead to a high calorie intake and the piling on of those pounds.

So, instead of turning to food when you feel unloved, find new activities to get involved in. Think about what you enjoy doing and arrange to go out and take part in these activities. This way you'll meet others who share your interests, you'll make some great new friends and possibly even find a new lover if that's what you desire. Don't let shyness or fear get in the way either, or the fact that you have no one to hold your hand; there are plenty of things it's socially acceptable to do on your own. You could try:

❖ A dance group — ceroc, rock and roll, Latin American.

❖ Yoga or meditation classes.

❖ Helping out at school or playgroup.

❖ A night class.

❖ Joining a gym.

❖ Self-defence classes.

❖ Joining (or forming) a book club.

Whatever takes your fancy is fine; you just need to stay occupied, get out and meet new friends, and have a good time.

Eating in Secret
We've all done it, bought that forbidden chocolate bar and sneakily eaten it out of view. After all, if no one saw you eat it, you can pretend it didn't happen. Why do we do this? Perhaps it's because we feel people will judge us,

because we feel that what we are doing is inherently wrong, and because we want to be perceived as successful, motivated and in control. Eating chocolate when you're on a diet might show you were unsuccessful, unmotivated and out of control in your own eyes!

Eating in secret can lead to feelings of guilt and low self-esteem in the longer term, and you can really put weight on this way. It's a difficult habit to break but you can look at strategies for overcoming the problem.

Talk to your friends, and gain their perspective. Let people know that you're not on a strict diet but a healthy eating regimen where high-calorie foods are eaten as occasional treats. Once you've given yourself permission to eat 'naughty foods', and informed others of this, you won't feel so guilty and you won't feel judged. Cut down slowly if you eat large amounts in secret. Set yourself achievable goals, which you can aim for gradually, rather than trying to make extreme changes overnight.

This is a hard habit to break, but you can do it with support and understanding.

Stress
The pressures today on how we perform and how we look are immense. The perfect woman is perceived to have a successful career, a husband whom she helps and supports, and children who are polite, well groomed and well adjusted. Not only that, but we are expected to look young, slim and glamorous. A lack of achievement in any area can be viewed as failure by women themselves, by family and friends, and by society as a whole. Even for men these days life is getting more stressful; they are expected to pull their weight at home and can no longer just go out to work and expect to come home to dinner on the table and their slippers warming by the fire.

Being pulled in all directions can cause a considerable amount of stress, and one of the ways we cope is by seeking release in food. Usually we just reach for the nearest convenient food, which is often a chocolate bar, sweets or biscuits. Have you noticed too that often you don't even taste or notice what you're eating? Sometimes it can be quite a shock to realise that you've polished off a packet of biscuits while you were fretting.

If you recognise that stress is making you overeat, you can address the underlying problem. Stress often occurs when we have too much to do and feel we are losing control of our lives. It might be that you're trying to hold down a high-pressure, full-time job, as well as keeping on top of all the housework, making sure the house is stocked up with food, looking after the children – the list goes on. If you feel you are losing control, it's time to sit back and take stock. Is there anything you can do to get better organised? Is there anyone else who can help you – family, partner, friends, neighbours? Can you cut down your hours at work, or possibly get a cleaner to take some pressure off at home?

Often we are so busy we put our own needs last, after everyone else's. It's important to have some 'you' time, whether this is half an hour each morning with a meditation tape, a couple of trips a week to the gym, or even a facial once a week. Have a look at the list of ideas here.

Pampering Yourself

❖ Read a book.   ❖ Meet a friend for coffee.

❖ Have a glass of wine.   ❖ Have a sleep.

❖ Have a foot bath or bubble bath.   ❖ Have a massage.

❖ Dye your hair or do your nails.   ❖ Pick some flowers.

❖ Light a candle.   ❖ Sit and be still.

❖ Dance around the house.   ❖ Take a walk in the countryside.

❖ Go to the movies.

Don't take yourself too seriously all the time: have some real fun! Find out about relaxation techniques in Chapter 11, or try yoga or meditation.

PROBLEM EATING

Although you may control your food intake very well while on a diet, once you slip up and eat something that's not on the diet, you may think, 'Oh, what the hell, I've broken the diet now so I may as well really go for it and eat what I like. I can always start again tomorrow.' Rather than just an extra couple of hundred calories you might find yourself having an extra couple of thousand calories.

If you recognise this behaviour in yourself, you really need to try and break the habit. Here are a few tips:

❖ Make sure you aren't too hard on yourself with the regimen you're following; include some of your favourite treats.

❖ Understand it's the overall balance that's important. Accept that you are entitled to occasional biscuits and other treats.

❖ Don't get angry with yourself if you eat something you think you shouldn't have – we're all human! Learn from your mistakes; don't chastise yourself over them.

❖ Reassure yourself that you don't need to binge.

❖ Solve the problem. If you're eating in response to a particular situation, try to deal with that rather than seeking solace in food.

❖ If you really need to eat, keep some healthy snacks on hand. Fruit and vegetables are always good – pick your favourites and go for dried, frozen, and tinned as well as fresh.

❖ Plan ahead. If an activity is coming up where you know you could overeat, plan some distractions.

❖ Use the support of others. There's nothing like talking to a group of friends who have been through the same sorts of experiences.

OVERCOMING SETBACKS

So what do you do if you've had a complete blow-out? You have consumed everything within your reach in a feeding frenzy and now you feel disgusting. You may be feeling guilt and regret; you may be wondering how you could possibly have done this to yourself. You may feel like just giving up!

It is important to be kind to yourself. Recognise you are a human being with frailties and not some pre-programmed robot. Remember that this is just one small segment of your life; it isn't the end of the world. Do something nice for yourself in order to move away from the feeling of self-blame; perhaps take a walk, read a book or watch a video, something that will take your mind off things. Share the problem with an understanding and compassionate friend. Sharing this kind of thing is the first step in taking away the power that food has over your life.

Once you feel ready, think about what triggered you to binge eat; there might be many causes (see Emotional Reasons for Eating on page 31). Think about what you might do next time you are feeling this way, or are in the same situation again. Think how you could alter your actions and make a different choice other than eating. Treat the experience as a learning experience.

THE POWER OF THE MIND

The mind is a powerful tool. It affects how we feel about ourselves, our weight and how we tackle issues around food. Now we've had a look at some key reasons for eating and ways to take the focus off food, we'll address the issue of what being fat means for you, assess your current frame of mind, and suggest ways to change old patterns of behaviour.

THE MEANING OF YOUR WEIGHT

In her book *Fat is a Feminist Issue*,[2] psychotherapist Susie Orbach looks at reasons why people are fat and suggests that it is not possible to lose weight until you have understood the fundamental question, 'What is the meaning of your fat to you?' She suggests that to be fat is to have a security blanket or defence between you and the rest of the world, as the illustration opposite shows, and that women who are overweight actually have an interest in being so. Initially this may sound far-fetched. After all, we live in a society that is prejudiced against the fatter person, so why would anyone want to be fat?

However, sometimes an extra layer can seem to protect us from the outside world. Being physically big can make you feel strong, and better able to handle bullying, for example. It can also give you a reason not to live your life to the full, telling yourself, 'I won't go to that party, I'm too fat', or 'I can't apply for that job, they'll judge me on my appearance'. You have a valid excuse not to put yourself into any social situation that you might find difficult or challenging, even if you were not overweight. You can also use your fat to procrastinate, convincing yourself that you do intend to make changes, while remaining in your comfort zone: 'I'll start going to the pool once I've lost some weight.' For some, there is a subconscious desire to remain fat in order to be insulated from the risks and unpredictability of a fuller life.

However, if you did become thinner, you could no longer make these excuses. This may be why some of us may indulge in food as a way of saying 'stuff you' to the world. The irony is, however, that you are only really 'stuffing up' yourself, in terms of your future health and happiness.

A lifelong approach to weight loss involves not only addressing your eating habits and activity levels but also some of the emotional and psychological issues. Enlist the support of your friends and family and do get involved in meeting people. Support is one of the key ways of getting into a new routine that results in sustained changes to your life.

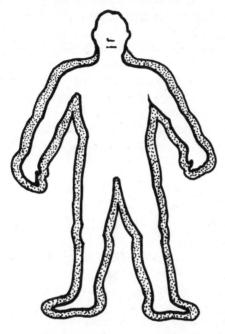

Extra pounds: a security blanket of fat protecting a person's spiritual, intellectual and emotional core self.

UNDERSTANDING BEHAVIOUR CHANGE

Changing your behaviour is a widely used strategy in treating weight problems. One approach was developed about 20 years ago after researchers compared the success of people who had given up smoking on their own with those involved in treatment programmes.[3] Smoking is highly addictive and giving up can be an immense challenge. It is now recognised that some of the theories that apply to giving up smoking can also be applied to changing dietary habits. Distinct stages have been identified, and these are outlined on pages 42–43.

The Behaviour Change Process Explained

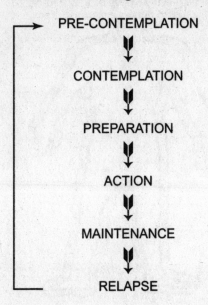

PRE-CONTEMPLATION

⇓

CONTEMPLATION

⇓

PREPARATION

⇓

ACTION

⇓

MAINTENANCE

⇓

RELAPSE

PRE-CONTEMPLATION When you are at this stage you are not considering making any changes to your life or your eating habits for the foreseeable future. We all know people who are at this stage; maybe they are happy with their weight, or they are unable to change, but whatever the reason for not wanting to change, people at this stage have no intention of doing anything about it.

CONTEMPLATION As you are reading this book it is very likely you are at the stage of contemplating making some changes. You are considering whether to make a change: can you really do it? Is it possible? How would you go about it? You are not yet actually ready to make the changes in your life that are needed but thinking about it is obviously a very important first step. If this is where you are at currently, think about moving on to the next stage, preparation.

PREPARATION When you are preparing to make changes, you have made an actual commitment to yourself to instigate a change. You are busy getting together the knowledge and skills needed to make the change. This may include reading a book such as this one to understand how you can get the changes in place in your life to lose weight and keep it off for ever. It is likely you have tried to make changes previously in your life so have made some small changes already. Perhaps you are eating a bit more fruit, a bit less fat, are exercising a little. You are probably planning to make changes in the near future, say over the next month or so, and you are committed to putting changes in place.

ACTION This is the stage where you are actually beginning to put in place those changes. You have read this book and have developed a lifelong strategy to lose weight, to eat a healthier diet and to get fit. You have a plan in place and are beginning to follow this plan. You are well on the way to success.

MAINTENANCE The changes in your lifestyle and eating habits are now becoming well established and integrated. It is no longer new and different; you have probably lost quite a significant amount of weight by now and are finding things quite straightforward. You are probably about six months into becoming a new you.

RELAPSE This is where you have fallen over. The changes have not been possible to maintain. Maybe you tried to do too much too soon and it wasn't sustainable. If this is the case you need to start again at the pre-contemplation stage and this time move more slowly through the stages, making changes much more gradually. Maybe there was an event in your life that was incredibly stressful – a new job, a divorce, a new baby – and the last thing on your mind was sticking to the new diet and lifestyle habits you had established successfully. Take some time out for you to recover, and then begin again slowly. Don't give up – you are too important for that, and just think about all the benefits to your health and your life in the longer term.

The first thing for you to do is to have a look at this model for change and figure out where you are up to. Have you no intention of making any changes (unlikely as you are reading this book)? Are you just thinking about it? Have you actually started the preparations for change? Are you making the changes? Are you managing to sustain the new lifestyle? Have you fallen into a relapse situation? Once you have figured out where you are at, then you need to move forwards onto the next area of change for you. Don't worry if you have to start at the beginning; just get yourself in the right frame of mind, understand where you are at and use this book to plan out and implement the changes that are going to give you a whole new life.

If you are just thinking about getting ready to make changes or are in the planning stages it can be helpful not only to have the courage to admit there is an issue but also to seek help and support from others by sharing problems and seeking solutions. Part of the philosophy underpinning the power of positive eating is that you need support to succeed, whether it be from a health professional such as a dietitian, from friends or family or even from your pet – you can take a new puppy for a walk. For now, though, an important first step to getting started is to understand the Steps of Courage you need to succeed.

STEPS OF COURAGE

If you are thinking about making changes, or are in the planning stages, bravo! You have the courage to admit there is a problem and you can now begin to move forwards through the seven steps of courage shown below.

1.	HAVE THE COURAGE	to admit you have a problem.
2.	BE HONEST	about the foods you eat and the lifestyle you lead, both to yourself and to others.
3.	SHARE	your problems and issues, and offer and receive support to help you succeed.
4.	SEEK SOLUTIONS	to the problems and look at ways that you can implement changes that will help you succeed and that will fit into your lifestyle.
5.	GROW AND DEVELOP	as you learn new behaviours and sustain the changes in your life.
6.	BELIEVE IN YOURSELF	Think positively and know that you can succeed.
7.	BECOME	a new, fitter, healthier and happier person; share your successes with others to help them succeed too, leading by example.

Diets always begin tomorrow, so the saying goes, but there's no time like the present to start making changes that will be of such great benefit in the longer term. Remember, you aren't about to embark on some torturous regimen with physical activities you hate and none of the foods you enjoy. The trick is working out which changes in diet and activity will work for you. The starting point might be just to carry on as you are for a week while recording your feelings when you eat different foods. It might be, however, that you are keen to get straight into a whole new lifestyle. The important thing is to begin the changes now, and to ensure that they are easy, achievable, and enjoyable.

4

MAGICAL MYSTERY CURES

Dieting is certainly big business. If you're struggling with
your weight there is no end of options open to you, from
the credible through to the wacky! At your local library or
bookshop you'll find shelves full of titles offering to give
you back eternal youth, to guarantee that you will lose
weight if you follow their magic formula, to cleanse your
body of toxins – the list goes on. Miracle diet books are
certainly very believable. Often they use complex medical
jargon, which could dupe even the most astute reader.
There are also special foods, herbal preparations and even
plasters that are claimed to help you lose weight.

Some of the diets can work, but most are just a rip-off.
The effective diets work only because you are eating fewer
calories as you try and mix the odd combinations of food.
Even if they work in the short term, it is unlikely that a
peculiar eating pattern will be sustainable in the longer
term. When you return to your old eating habits, the inevi-
table happens. That's right, your weight piles back on again.

MISINFORMATION
In its 1995 position paper on Food and Nutrition Misinformation[1] the American Dietetic Association (ADA) defines
three areas that we should look out for as consumers:

❖ Food faddism: exaggerated claims are made for the
effect a particular food or diet can have, for example
the myth that low-carbohydrate diets can induce
weight loss.

❖   Food quackery: inaccurate information promoted by
    people who believe it is true, but who are themselves
    misguided.

❖   Health fraud: the deliberate promotion of inaccurate
    information for financial gain.

The advice from the ADA is buyer beware. More specifically we are advised to:

❖   Understand the concepts of food fads, food quackery
    and health fraud.

❖   Question the qualifications of the authors of differ-
    ent diets or food regimens.

❖   Look for evidence of effectiveness: is the diet sup-
    ported by good scientific studies published in sound
    journals, or are personal opinion and anecdotes used
    to sell the idea?

❖   Look for sound advice from a registered dietitian, or
    contact a local health department, hospital, or
    university.

A recent paper published by the US *FDA Consumer* magazine[2] gives advice on ways to spot a health fraud. Here are
some of the signs to look out for.

Personal Testimonials
*I lost heaps of weight without changing what I eat or taking
any exercise. If it worked for me it can work for you too.*

Often when there is no evidence to support a particular
product or diet you will see personal testimonials without
any scientific evidence to back these up. If a diet is making
wild and exaggerated claims and has only personal testimonials as evidence that it works, then be wary!

Quick Fix
Lose weight fast without dieting or exercise.

We've all seen these weight-loss solutions. Of course you

never have to put in any effort, just use the product, eat as much as you like and the weight will fall off. While some of us may want to believe this, let's face it: we know it doesn't really work! Don't waste your money.

Rapid Weight Loss
Lose a stone in just two weeks.

We all want to lose weight quickly and look good as soon as possible. But be wary of diets that promote rapid weight loss. The ideal amount of weight to lose safely is just 0.5–1kg (1–2 lb) a week. Substantial weight reduction will lead to a loss of lean tissue, which is undesirable. Also, you will initially be losing just glycogen (your body's carbohydrate store) and water, and as soon as you eat normally again you will just put the weight back on.

One Product Does it All
Try this diet for a younger, healthier, fitter, slimmer, more beautiful you.

Whatever your particular problem, this product will help: weight loss, muscle tone, looking younger, having more energy, feeling less stressed. When you see these types of claims on a product, be sceptical.

Spot-reducing
Big thighs? Spot-reduce weight from this part of your body with this new wonder diet.

Exploiting the fact that we all have a part of our body that we'd like to slim down, whether it's our hips, thighs, buttocks, upper arms or tummies, a number of diets claim to help you lose weight from a particular area. Don't be fooled: you can't spot-reduce by eating a particular combination of foods.

Boosting Your Metabolism
Lose weight fast on this brand new miracle diet that actually makes your metabolism work faster.

There are ways to help boost your metabolic rate and

burn up more calories; exercise is a really good one. However, eating certain foods won't boost your metabolism to such an extent that you will lose weight; it's the overall calorie intake that is important.

Natural
Naturally aids weight loss.

There are innumerable products that are claimed to be natural. Be careful, as there is an implication that they are safer than conventional treatments. A product that is natural is not necessarily safe or even effective. And remember that any product potent enough to work is potent enough to have side-effects.

Satisfaction Guaranteed
Money-back guarantee, full refund given.

Money-back guarantees are often promised if you don't lose weight. However, it's worth pointing out that the marketers of fraudulent products rarely stay in one place for long. As their customers are unlikely to find them, they can afford to be generous with their guarantees.

Time Tested
Ancient remedy, used for thousands of years.

Be wary of claims on products that are said to be 'ancient remedies', or 'based on folklore'. This doesn't necessarily mean that they actually work, or indeed that they are safe.

Meaningless Medical Jargon
Scientifically proven thermoregulatory thermogenesis effect on genetically or phenotypically pre-set conditions with sympathomimetic and stimulant properties.

A complicated jumble of medical terminology, such as we've concocted here, is often used to promote miracle cures. The aim is to confuse people, but these fanciful terms usually cover up the fact that there is no evidence the diet works. Even if the promoters quote scientific studies, the chance that most people will actually go and look up the paper is pretty slim; that's how they get away with it!

WHO'S WHO IN THE NUTRITION WORLD
It's also mightily confusing trying to sift through the fact and the fiction when it comes to advice on nutrition. Who do you believe? How do you distinguish the experts from the quacks? You need to look at who is giving the advice and what their qualifications are.

Registered Dietitians
Registered dietitians will have undertaken a degree course at university and trained in hospital and community settings. They will be registered with a body that monitors standards and fitness to practise, such as a Health Professions Council or a Dietitians' Board. Dietitians can give advice on dietary requirements, and recommend appropriate food intakes for both the healthy population and those with particular diseases or conditions. Registered dietitians are a credible source of information on food and nutrition.

Registered Nutritionists
Schemes are currently set up in some countries to register nutritionists who have a relevant degree and a high level of experience. Look out for the words 'registered nutritionist', and contact the relevant nutrition society for a list of who is registered.

Doctors
General practitioners and other medical doctors may give advice on general nutrition, although they will usually refer patients with conditions that require specialist dietary advice to a registered dietitian.

Individuals who have studied for a PhD may go by the title of 'Doctor', even though they could be qualified in anything from rocket science to sociology. It doesn't necessarily mean they are qualified in medicine or indeed nutrition.

Nutrition Experts, Health Gurus and Certified Instructors
Unqualified people may call themselves a whole host of names, and self-appointed nutrition experts, health gurus and certified instructors abound. Always ask about their qualifications. Do they have a recognised degree qualification in nutrition or dietetics? Are they a member of a professional organisation or registered with a board or authority? Or have they simply spent the odd afternoon at the library, or done a course lasting a few days or weeks, gaining a meaningless certificate?

POPULAR DIETS
Let's have a look at some of the diets on offer and see which ones are likely to work and which are just plain silly.

Low-carbohydrate Diets
These diets involve cutting down on carbohydrates such as bread, rice, potatoes and pasta, and cutting down on some fruits and vegetables. It is a concept that has been around for many years. Some of the proponents of this type of diet have suggested it can help weight loss by giving the body a 'metabolic advantage' over more conventional diets. There is, however, no evidence to support this concept; any weight lost will be down to eating fewer calories rather than any magic effect of avoiding carbohydrates.

In fact, in the short term, these diets cause a greater loss of body water than body fat, and when the diet ends, water weight is re-gained[3].

A paper published by the American Heart Association[4] advises against high-protein, low-carbohydrate diets because they restrict healthy foods that provide essential nutrients and do not provide the variety of foods that are needed to meet nutritional needs adequately.

Studies published in 2003 in the *New England Journal of*

Medicine[5,6] found that people on low-carbohydrate diets did lose weight over a six-month period, however much of the weight was re-gained again after a year[5]. Even the authors of these studies say that further research is needed to evaluate the long-term safety and effectiveness of such diets.

The reason dietitians don't generally recommend these diets is because they don't seem to work in the longer term, because they can be associated with unpleasant side-effects and because for some people they may actually be harmful. The very-low-carbohydrate diets are inadvisable for the following reasons:

❖   Depriving the body of carbohydrates can lead to a condition called ketosis; the side-effects of ketosis are weakness, nausea, dehydration, diminished energy and bad breath. You'll probably feel pretty grumpy once you are in this state and the consequences could be serious for people with diabetes.

❖   Much of the initial weight loss is down to loss of the body's carbohydrate stores (glycogen) and water loss.

❖   This type of diet is very prescriptive and not easily sustainable in the long term. Although weight loss may occur, it is likely that it will be re-gained once old eating habits are resumed.

❖   There is likely to be inadequate variety in the foods eaten and therefore nutritional intake might be compromised. In particular, fibre intakes are likely to be low as fibre is found in wholegrain cereal foods. Also, intake of some vitamins and minerals is likely to be low.

❖   It can be excessively high in fat, saturated fatty acids and cholesterol. High-fat diets have been linked to heart disease and some types of cancer. There is a need for more research on the effect of this diet on cardio-vascular risk, especially during weight maintenance.

❖   The level of protein is high. Excess intake of protein is undesirable for people with diabetes as it can put strain on the kidneys; diabetics should consult a registered dietitian for the most appropriate advice. More research is needed into the effects of low-carbohydrate diets on long-term kidney function.

❖   A very low intake of carbohydrate means that exercise may be difficult. We need some carbohydrate stores for energy when we exercise for any length of time.

❖   The long-term consequences on health and the safety of the low-carbohydrate diets for those with serious obesity-related diseases are as yet unknown.

❖   More research is certainly needed on this type of dietary regimen before firm recommendations can be made about long-term safety and effectiveness.

Overall, there are no good scientific data to support the low-carbohydrate diets and these regimens contradict the nutrition advice from authoritative government and non-government organisations throughout the world.

Food Combinations
Dr William Hay developed the food-combining diet in the early 1900s. More recently it has re-emerged and a number of books advocating this approach have achieved great popularity. The theory is that you shouldn't eat carbohydrate foods (starches such as bread or rice, and sugars such as table sugar) at the same time as protein foods. Five rules are set out:

❖   Do not eat starches and sugars at the same time as proteins and acid fruits.

❖   Vegetables, salads and fruits should form the major part of the diet.

❖   Eat protein, starch and fat in small quantities.

❖   Eat only wholegrain and unprocessed starches. Avoid all refined and processed foods.

❖   Allow at least four hours between meals of different types.

Proponents of this diet claim that the digestive system works more effectively and that you will achieve weight loss and improved health and well-being. This approach certainly won't do you any harm. You may even lose some weight as you grapple with the complex meal arrangements, and try to make them appetising. Also, it's based on fruit, vegetables and wholegrains, which we all know are good for us. The down side is as follows:

❖   There is absolutely no scientific evidence to support the concept. All the books are supported only by testimonials and anecdotes. Our bodies are, in fact, perfectly capable of digesting any combination of foods we may wish to consume.

❖   It's difficult to follow, and meals are unlikely to be appetising or interesting.

❖   In the longer term it's impossible to stick to.

❖   Any weight loss is due to a lower energy intake. In fact, you can achieve this with a sensible balanced diet (see Chapter 5).

The expert verdict on this one: don't waste your time, effort or money.

Crash Diets
They're ever-popular for getting slim for that all-important holiday or wedding, but does the tempting crash diet really work? The simple answer is 'no'. If it means having fewer than 800 kcal a day, it is actually harmful as there would be a significant loss of lean body tissue. Other drawbacks are:

❖ Much of the weight lost will not be fat, but glycogen (carbohydrate stores in the body) mixed with water.

❖ As soon as you begin to eat normally and replenish your carbohydrate and water stores, the weight will return.

❖ Rapid loss of weight is almost always followed by weight gain, so it's a waste of time! Also, it can increase the risk of gallstones.[7]

Blood-group Diets
This is truly one of the more weird approaches. The theory is that you should follow a particular diet depending on what blood group you are:[8]

❖ Type O: eat meat and steer clear of wheat and most other grains.

❖ Type A: have a vegetarian diet.

❖ Type B: have a varied diet that includes meat. This is supposed to be the only blood type that does well with dairy products.

❖ Type AB: these are said to 'have most of the benefits and intolerances of types A and B'.

This theory is seriously flawed and there is no scientific evidence to back it. There is a very high risk of ending up with a diet that is poorly balanced, or even deficient in some important nutrients. What's more, it would be pretty boring following some of the restrictive regimens.

Zone Diets
Dietary recommendations for this method include:

❖ Eat rigid quantities of food at specific times for proportionate sources of energy: 40 per cent of energy from carbohydrate, 30 per cent of energy from protein and 30 per cent of energy from fat.

❖   Divide meals and snacks into blocks of protein (7g each), blocks of carbohydrate (9g each), and blocks of fat (3g each).

❖   At each meal women should eat about three blocks each of fat, protein and carbohydrate, and men about four blocks.

❖   Meals should be no more than 500 kcal, and snacks no more than 100 kcal.

❖   It is suggested that maintaining this rigid balance will control certain hormone levels in a tight 'zone', so helping weight loss.

It is claimed that to 'enter the zone' is to enter a state of exceptional health well known to champion athletes, and that not only will your body burn fat, but it will fight heart disease, diabetes, PMS, chronic fatigue, depression and cancer. Wild claims indeed, but with no good scientific evidence to support them.

Although the zone diet is not as extreme as some of the low-carbohydrate regimens, it is complex and would be difficult for most dieters to follow for any period. The level of carbohydrate is less than that recommended by health experts and is, therefore, not particularly good for long-term health. The metabolic theories are flawed and not in line with current knowledge in the fields of nutrition, biochemistry and physiology. This one is best avoided.

Liver-cleansing Diet
The theory behind the liver-cleansing diet is that excess weight and a sluggish metabolism are a result of an unhealthy liver. The eight-week 'liver-cleansing' plan involves following a gentle regimen for two weeks, followed by four weeks of a more serious cleansing plan, then a return to a less demanding plan for another two weeks.

Recommended foods include raw fruit and vegetables, legumes, seeds, nuts, fish, free-range chicken and eggs. Red meat is kept to a minimum and the advice is to avoid dairy products.

The truth of the matter is that this short-term diet will do little actually to cleanse the liver and there is no evidence that a poorly functioning liver leads to weight gain. Also, if you avoid dairy products, your calcium levels could be reduced, and there is no evidence that meat has any adverse effect on the liver. However, the diet is based on healthy foods; fruits, vegetables and legumes are good for anyone, including those who are aiming to lose weight.

Detox Diets
The idea behind detox diets is that periodically we need to clear the 'toxic waste' from our bodies in order to stay healthy. It is also claimed that we can magically lose weight by detoxifying our bodies. Detox diets often last from one day to one month and may involve:

❖   Complete fasting.

❖   Eating just fruit and vegetables.

❖   Restricting food intake to avoid such foods as wheat and dairy foods.

❖   Avoidance of caffeine, alcohol and refined foods.

The fact is, if the human body really accumulated lots of toxins, then we would feel ill. The concept of detox diets is irrational and unscientific. When you starve your body of calories you build up chemicals called ketones. These chemicals (as previously mentioned) can result in nausea, dehydration, weakness, light-headedness and irritability.

As with crash diets, any rapid weight loss is likely to be regained once you start eating properly again.

With regard to advice to avoid wheat and dairy products, for most of us this is unnecessary and could potentially be harmful as these foods provide an important source of nutrients. For those with a true allergy to milk, wheat, or any other food, the condition should be diagnosed by a qualified medical practitioner and managed under the supervision of a registered dietitian. It does make sense to avoid excessive intakes of caffeine, alcohol and high-fat, high-sugar foods, however, fasting or severely restricting food consumption limits the intake of energy and important nutrients that are needed for health and well-being.

Zen Macrobiotics
The philosophy of this diet is based on the principles of yin and yang (negative and positive respectively) for optimum spiritual, mental and physical well-being. It involves a progression through ten levels, from a diet that is fairly well balanced to one consisting only of cereals. At this extreme the diet could actually be quite dangerous, as it's severely deficient in some nutrients.

Cabbage Soup or Grapefruit …
We've all come across the one-food-only diet, where we are told that eating copious amounts of a particular food will magically help us lose those extra pounds. While living solely on these foods will certainly help reduce your intake of calories, there is nothing magical about this. What's more, you won't be able to stick to them for very long and they won't be very enjoyable.

Sweating it Out
Some people believe that a good way to lose weight is to spend lots of time in a sauna or steam room to 'sweat off' the extra weight. You may lose some weight this way, but it will be just fluids and not fat. As soon as you have a drink you will just put it back on.

Pills, Potions and Plasters
There are certainly some bizarre gimmicks for weight loss. Pills, potions, even plasters have been touted as the latest

magical remedy for weight loss, to dissolve away that excess fat. Needless to say there is no evidence that they work, and some herbal preparations could even be harmful. Before taking tablets of this type, always check with your doctor or dietitian.

BUT THERE MUST BE A MAGIC SOLUTION

There is an easy solution to weight loss. It certainly doesn't involve following all sorts of funny combinations and permutations of food intake, although these types of regimens will be so difficult to follow they will probably lead to weight loss as you will be eating less. It's got nothing to do with any magical physiological effects, or any amazing metabolic boosting effects; it's just that reduction in energy intake. The simple solution is to reduce calorie intake and increase exercise. The challenge exists in putting this into practice, but that's where we can help you with our whole-body, whole-lifestyle approach. Understanding the ins and outs of all the complex jargon that's about is certainly useful, but now we need to concentrate on the real solutions that will help you achieve that goal of losing weight and keeping it off.

The dietary solution to long-term weight loss and maintenance of that weight loss is all pretty straight-forward. You just need to follow a few basic rules in terms of what you eat:

❖ Eat plenty of wholegrain carbohydrate foods such as cereals, wholemeal bread and brown rice and pasta.

❖ Eat lots of fruits and vegetables as snacks, with meals, and as desserts.

❖ Consume moderate amounts of iron-containing foods such as lean meat, fish, pulses and nuts.

❖ Consume moderate amounts of calcium-containing foods such as low-fat milk, yoghurt and low-fat cheese.

❖ Limit your intake of fatty and sugary foods to the occasional treat.

❖ Ensure your portion sizes are appropriate.

Any diet that is based on these good solid principles of healthy eating will help you lose weight and maintain good health in the longer term, so just evaluate carefully yourself what's on offer. Have a look at the following chapters for some sensible information on what sort of foods to eat.

5

A BALANCED DIET: WHAT'S IT ALL ABOUT?

In the next three chapters we'll take a look at some basic nutrition principles and definitions, a new way of eating and living, and some food and meal solutions. The philosophy behind the power of positive eating is one of balance and moderation in terms of foods. It is all about modifying your own eating habits to lose weight, and then sustain the weight loss in the longer term. That's why you won't find long lists of foods or meals that you have to eat on a particular day. Dietary regimens that encourage you to eat a predetermined list of foods are unlikely to work in the long term, as you won't be able to stick to them for ever. It is much better to use your current diet as a starting point and to modify this to make it healthier.

This type of food pattern will fit well with your family situation and lifestyle so is much more likely to work. It is suitable not just for those who are overweight, but for everyone, to optimise health status and to reduce risk of chronic disease later in life.

Calorie counting is to be discouraged; the best philosophy is to aim for a balanced and varied diet, based on lots of wholegrains, fruits and vegetables, which is low in fat. Advice will be given on how to use the food group approach and on reasonable portion sizes. Also, it is important to remember there are no good or bad foods; it is the overall balance of the diet that is important, so if you want to eat chips and chocolate you can, as long as it is only as an occasional treat and forms a small proportion of your diet, as discussed later in this chapter.

RATE OF WEIGHT LOSS

Most people want to lose weight as quickly as possible: that's why the fad diets and instant cures are so popular (see Chapter 4). However, if you want to maintain that loss, you need realistic goals and an eating pattern that you can stick to.

Aim to shed 0.25–1kg per week (0.5–2 lb), which is equivalent to 13–52kg per year (2–8 stone), until you reach your target weight. This is slower than many people would like, but remember you are probably reducing weight much faster than you gained it in the first place.

EATING PATTERNS

Many diets recommend a particular eating pattern as a way of increasing the metabolic rate and, therefore, helping weight loss. Some authors propose eating lots of small meals; others advise three main meals in a day. But who is right?

The scientific research into this area suggests that the meal patterns you adopt have very little effect on your metabolic rate. It is unlikely that they affect your weight either up or down.

The best advice is to do what suits you, your family situation and your lifestyle. If you like to have lots of small snacks and light meals, that's just fine. If you prefer to have just three meals a day and nothing in between, that's okay too. The most important consideration is the overall food intake throughout the day, so don't be drawn into a change just because it's the latest fad.

BASIC NUTRITION

Most of us who have watched our weight have a fairly good understanding of basic nutrition. However, there can sometimes be some confusion over the more complex terms. Most of us like to work with calories, for example, as a measure of energy, but on some food labels energy values may be given as kilojoules. 'What's the difference?' you may ask. Well, this is explained below. Also, you may find information on the different types of fatty acids useful, which ones are better, how many calories in each. The following guide runs through in simple terms some basic nutrition facts that are useful for anyone following a weight-reducing regimen or simply looking to have a healthy diet.

Energy

We get energy from food. Our bodies use it for activity, or store it. Different units can be used for energy values. The most popular unit is the kilocalorie (kcal) (sometimes known as the Calorie). The term used on food labels is kilojoule (kJ), although kcal may be given as well.

In order to convert kJ into kcal, use the following formula:

kcal = kJ divided by 4.2

In other words, a kcal has roughly a quarter of the value of a kJ.

As a guide, the average daily energy requirement for a woman is about 2000 kcal, and for a man about 2500 kcal. It is important to remember that these are just average figures and do not apply to everyone. A petite and inactive woman will have a much lower energy requirement than one who is tall and active. However, if you reduce your daily energy intake to 500–1000 kcal below requirements, this should result in a weight loss of 0.5–1kg (1–2 lb) per week.

Carbohydrates

At least half of our energy intake should be provided by carbohydrate foods. Reducing the amount of fat in the diet and increasing the proportion of carbohydrate is likely to reduce energy intake, as carbohydrate provides, on a weight-for-weight basis, about half as many calories as fat.

There is no scientific evidence to support the low-carbohydrate, high-fat diets as a way of losing weight; in fact they can even be dangerous (see Chapter 4). However, a diet high in unrefined carbohydrates can have a positive impact on health, particularly for those at risk of excess weight, heart disease, adult-onset diabetes and some types of cancer. This was confirmed in a recent paper on strategies for weight management.[1] Carbohydrates can be divided into starch and sugars.

Starches

Starchy foods include potatoes, bread, breakfast cereals, rice and pasta. These should be the main sources of energy in our diets; they also provide B vitamins, and wholegrain varieties provide dietary fibre. It is important to avoid adding too much fat to carbohydrate foods (for example, butter in potatoes, potato chips that are fried, butter on bread). Stay away from high-fat breads such as croissants, and have pitta or a bread roll instead. Wholegrain varieties can help to fill you up.

Sugars

Sugar is a general term for a number of sweet-tasting substances including sucrose (table sugar), fructose (fruit sugar), lactose (milk sugar) and glucose. If you have a sweet tooth, there is no harm in including a little sugar in your diet – for example, a scraping of jam on your toast or the occasional dessert. If you do wish to have sugary treats, have them as part of a meal and brush your teeth afterwards. Sucking sweets or drinking high-sugar beverages constantly throughout the day can have an adverse effect on your teeth and can push up your energy intake.

Dietary Fibre

Fibre is an important component of a healthy diet; it keeps your digestive system working properly and helps to prevent problems such as constipation.

Fibre can be found in foods such as wholegrain cereals

(e.g. bread, rice and pasta), legumes and other vegetables and fruits.

We should aim to have a diet that is based on wholegrain cereals, fruits and vegetables for optimal health.

Protein

Protein is needed for the growth and repair of body tissues. Protein-containing foods include meat, fish, eggs, milk and cheese. Protein can also be found in non-animal foods such as cereals, pulses and nuts, which are particularly useful sources for those on a vegan diet.

Most of us eat plenty of protein, so beware of the fad diets that promote high intakes. Also, watch out for any fat that may accompany a high-protein food; choose lean meat or cut off and discard all the fat, and choose low-fat dairy products.

Fat

We need a small amount of fat in our diets to provide fat-soluble vitamins and essential fatty acids, but many of us eat far more fat than we actually need. This is the number-one nutrient to target for reduction. Weight-for-weight, fat contains twice as many calories as carbohydrate, and all types of fat, whether saturated or unsaturated, contain the same number of calories. Just by adding fat to food it is possible to double the calorie content.

Some people are concerned that cutting down on fat could leave them deficient in essential fatty acids. In fact, this is almost impossible, as such small amounts are actually required. So the focus should certainly be to cut down on fat for optimal health and weight loss.

Not only is it important to reduce total fat intake, but you should also consider the types of fatty acids in your diet. An explanation of these, and their sources, is given below.

Saturated Fatty Acids

These can raise the level of cholesterol in the blood, increasing the risk of heart disease. Fats that are hard tend to contain a higher proportion of saturated fatty acids. The main sources include:

❖ Animal fats such as butter, lard, hard margarine, cheese, chicken skin and meat fat.

❖ Pies, pastries, potato crisps, cakes and biscuits.

❖ Palm oil and coconut oil.

Trans Fatty Acids
Trans fatty acids are produced during food processing, for example of hard margarines. We consume smaller amounts of these fats than of saturated fatty acids. However, this type of fat can also raise cholesterol levels and so increase the risk of heart disease; they should be kept to a minimum in the diet. Sources of trans fatty acids include:

❖ Hard margarines.

❖ Cakes, pastries and biscuits.

❖ Beef, lamb, milk and dairy fat.

Monounsaturated Fatty Acids
Monounsaturated fatty acids are a healthier form of fat, and can be used to replace the saturated fatty acids. The main sources are olive oil and rapeseed (canola) oil. Look out for the fat spreads based on these oils. Other sources are nuts, lean meat, chicken, eggs and fish.

Polyunsaturated Fatty Acids
These are also a healthier form of fat. There are two types. Omega-6 helps to reduce blood cholesterol levels. The main sources are sunflower and soybean oil, soft margarines, nuts and seeds. Omega-3 helps to reduce the tendency of the blood to clot, and may help to protect against heart disease. The main sources of the omega-3 fatty acids are oily fish such as herring, mackerel, salmon and sardines.

Cutting Back
Your intake of saturated and trans fatty acids should be kept to a minimum. Always trim the fat from meat and remove the skin from chicken, choose lower-fat dairy products, and either avoid or eat only a very limited amount of pies, cakes, biscuits, and hard spreads such as butter, lard and hard margarine.

Don't forget that all types of fat contain the same number of calories. However, by changing from saturated and trans fatty acids to the mono- and polyunsaturated fatty acids, you will make your diet much healthier, and reduce the risk of raised cholesterol and heart disease. All the same, do remember that you should not be increasing your intake of fat or pouring excessive amounts of oil over your foods. Try some of these suggestions:

❖ Bake your own cakes using the healthier types of fat, or eliminate the fat altogether (see Chapter 7 for recipes).

❖ Choose low-fat spreads and oils based on mono- or polyunsaturated fatty acids.

❖ Use spray oils based on mono- and polyunsaturated fats, to minimise the amount of fat.

❖ Include at least two portions a week of oily fish.

Alcohol
Alcohol can be a significant source of calories. If you do drink, remember that in terms of health risk, women should drink on average no more than two to three units in a day and men no more than three to four (total weekly intake should be below 14 and 21 units respectively for women and men). We should, of course, have some alcohol-free days. Women who may become pregnant or who are pregnant are advised to avoid alcohol.

One unit is equal to half a pint of ordinary strength beer, lager or cider; one small glass of wine; one pub measure of spirits.

It's useful to know which drinks contain the most calories. The table gives you a rough guide.

The Energy Content of Common Drinks	
Drink	**Energy Content (kcal)**
Half a pint of beer	85
1 small glass of dry sherry	60
1 average glass of wine	85
1 shot of spirit	50
(Source: *McCance and Widdowson's The Composition of Foods*[2])	

Vitamins and Minerals

Vitamins and minerals are important for good health. A balanced diet should provide all the vitamins and minerals we need. The role they play, and common food sources, are listed here.

Vitamin/Mineral	Function	Sources
Vitamin A	Aids growth and development, immune function, night vision.	Liver, kidney, whole milk, margarine. Carotenoids found in carrots, red and orange fruit and dark green vegetables can be converted into vitamin A in the body.
Vitamin D	Important for healthy bones.	Oily fish, fortified foods such as margarine and breakfast cereals. Can also be produced by the body on exposure to sunlight.
Vitamin E	Acts as an antioxidant and is involved in immune function.	Vegetable oils, wholegrain cereals, dark green vegetables and nuts.

Vitamin/ Mineral	Function	Sources
Vitamin K	Needed for clotting of the blood. May also play a role in bone health.	Green leafy vegetables, some fruit, vegetable oils and cereals.
Vitamin B1 (thiamin)	Involved in metabolism.	Cereals and potatoes. Some in meat, poultry and nuts.
Vitamin B2 (riboflavin)	Involved in metabolism.	Milk and milk products, fortified cereals. Some in meat and meat products.
Vitamin B3 (niacin)	Involved in metabolism.	Meat and meat products, bread, fortified cereals, potatoes, milk and milk products.
Vitamin B6	Involved in metabolism.	Potatoes and breakfast cereals.
Vitamin B12	Involved in metabolism.	Only found naturally in foods of animal origin, e.g. meat, meat products and milk. Often added to breakfast cereals.
Folate (folic acid)	Involved in metabolism. Helps development of the neural tube in unborn babies.	Wholegrain cereals, liver, leafy green vegetables.
Vitamin C	Needed for wound healing, healthy skin, a healthy immune system. Helps the absorption of iron from vegetable sources.	Citrus fruit, berry fruit, salad vegetables, peppers, potatoes.
Iron	Needed for healthy red blood cells, growth and development in young children.	Red meat, fish, fortified cereals, pulses and nuts. Plant sources of iron are less well absorbed by the body, but vitamin C can help absorption.
Calcium	Needed for healthy strong bones and teeth.	Milk and dairy products, canned fish eaten with bones, fortified breads and cereals. Some found in pulses, green vegetables, dried fruit and nuts.

Antioxidants

Antioxidants have had a lot of coverage in the popular press, but what exactly do they do, and where can you find them? Well, they are substances that help to prevent oxidation reactions in the body. Oxidation reactions are thought to be linked to ageing and the development of chronic diseases such as cancer and heart disease. Some vitamins and minerals have antioxidant effects – for example, vitamin C, vitamin E and carotenoids (which are converted to vitamin A in the body), selenium, manganese, zinc and copper.

New research shows that there is a whole range of other chemicals in plants that may also have antioxidant activity in the body, for example flavonoids found in red wine, and some fruit and vegetables, and lycopene found in tomatoes.

It is important to remember that there are hundreds of chemicals in a piece of fruit or in a vegetable, in a particular amount and combination. Although we know that eating fruit and vegetables is beneficial, and that part of the effect may be the presence of antioxidants, we do not yet know enough to recommend taking antioxidant supplements. These may in fact have adverse effects, particularly at high doses. Until there is much more large-scale research on humans, the current advice is to eat lots of fruit and vegetables and to stay away from high-dose antioxidant supplements.

Supplements

The use of vitamin and mineral supplements is increasing the world over, but are they really necessary? For most healthy people who have a balanced and varied diet, supplements are not necessary. There are some who may need some extra nutrients, for example:

❖   Women who might become pregnant, and pregnant women up to 12 weeks into their pregnancy, require folic acid supplements. Folic acid has been shown to reduce the risk of neural tube defects in the unborn baby.

❖ Women with high menstrual losses may need iron supplements.

❖ Anyone on a vegan or other restrictive diet may require supplements such as iron and vitamin B12.

Always ask for advice on supplements from your doctor or dietitian, and if you do decide to take them, follow the manufacturer's instructions. Avoid taking 'mega-doses' – quantities that are way in excess of recommended daily requirements.

THE FOOD-GROUP APPROACH
The food-group approach is used increasingly as a way of promoting the right food choices. This is the approach we would recommend you take as you embark on the power of positive eating regimen. The main principles are set out below.

Food Groups: How Much of Each?

❖ Lots of fruit and vegetables, which provide fibre and important vitamins and minerals. Aim for at least five portions a day (a portion is approximately a handful, but see Chapter 6 for more specific information).

❖ Lots of bread, cereals and potatoes, which provide energy, especially wholegrain varieties.

❖ Moderate amounts of lean meat, fish, pulses and nuts, which provide iron.

❖ Moderate amounts of lower-fat milk and dairy foods, which provide calcium.

❖ Small amounts of foods containing fats and sugars.

There are a number of ways of showing the different amounts you need – you may have seen pyramids, pie charts and even rainbows! The balanced-plate model adopted in the UK, and shown here, is useful as you can see how your dinner plate should look. Of course, this isn't literally what you should eat just at dinner: as long as your diet over a day or so is roughly in these proportions you are likely to be getting all the nutrients you need for optimal health. This is much easier than trying to count calories or stick to rigid meal plans. You can adapt all your meals and snacks to fit with this overall pattern, and when dishing out meals, make sure that the meat is lean, or the dairy foods are low in fat and that these foods do not take up too much of the plate. Most of your plate should be filled with vegetables and starchy foods. It's all about getting the proportions right rather than eating much less.

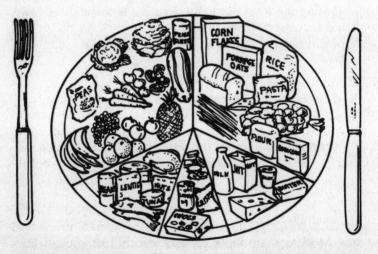

A balanced plate. From clockwise: bread, other cereals and potatoes; milk and dairy foods; foods containing fat, foods containing sugar; meat, fish and alternatives; fruit and vegetables.

Based on the Balance of Good Health, reproduced by kind permission of the Food Standards Agency, UK.

In Chapter 6 we discuss how much you need in each portion, and give you some suggestions for shopping and cooking.

GUIDELINES FOR A HEALTHY DIET
A few years ago the UK government devised eight guidelines for a healthy diet .[3] If you just remember these points you won't go far wrong.

Enjoy Your Food
This is the number one rule! We can sometimes forget when we are trying to alter our eating habits that food should be enjoyed; eating is one of the great pleasures in life! Look at ways of incorporating the foods you like. If your favourites are high in fat, just have them as an occasional treat, or look at adapting them to reduce the fat content.

Eat a Variety
By having lots of different foods in your diet, it's likely that you will get all the nutrients you need for good health.

Eat the Right Amount to be a Healthy Weight
When you are aiming to lose weight, do so gradually by eating the right sorts of foods. Be aware of the portion sizes and look at ways of reducing the fat in your food. More information on these areas is given in Chapters 6 and 7.

Eat Plenty of Foods Rich in Starch and Fibre
Most of our energy should come from these foods. Go for potatoes, wholegrain rice and pasta with main meals and avoid adding extra fat. Have wholegrain breakfast cereals, toast and pitta bread as snacks throughout the day.

Eat Plenty of Fruit and Vegetables
Aim to have at least five portions of fruit or vegetables throughout the day. They make great snacks, desserts and

accompaniments to main meals.

Don't Eat Too Many Foods That Contain a Lot of Fat
Be aware of the major sources of fat in the diet and focus on reducing your fat intake as a way of reducing your calorie intake. Fats are a concentrated source of calories.

Don't Have Sugary Foods Too Often
In particular, avoid having lots of high-sugar drinks or sugary sweets, as this can really pile on the extra calories without you realising it.

If You Drink Alcohol, Drink Sensibly
Alcohol is a source of energy, so drink in moderation, extend drinks with low-calorie mixers and lots of ice, and follow the guidelines for consumption outlined earlier.

In addition to the above guidelines, we should make sure that we don't have too much salt in our diet. Eating too much salt has been linked to high blood pressure, which may lead to an increased risk of heart disease and stroke. It is recommended that as adults we reduce our average intake of salt to around 6g a day. Avoid adding salt during cooking or at the table and avoid eating too many salty foods. Foods high in salt include snacks such as crisps and nuts, and salted foods such as bacon, cheese, pickles, smoked fish and many processed convenience meals.

6

NEW CHOICES, NEW HABITS

Now we have had a look at some basic nutrition and balanced eating principles in Chapter 5, we'll move on to look at new choices and new habits; from shopping and food preparation to cooking and eating. We'll also take a look at some common food myths and look at some real facts when it comes to food.

SHOPPING
Buying the right foods is a basic first step in establishing a new pattern of eating. Then by preparing and cooking these foods so that the fat content is minimised and the balance is right, you can be confident that you are on the road to success.

However, it's all too easy to buy the wrong things in the supermarket, with the aisles full of tempting products and packets. At this time, more than any other, it's important to be disciplined and to buy the right foods. Here are a few basic tips that can help you with your shopping.

❖ Never shop when you are hungry; this will just lead you to buy all the wrong foods.

❖ Always make a shopping list, and try to stick to it.

❖ If you have a real weakness for a particular food (such as chocolate, potato chips or cheese) to the extent that you know that you will just binge on it, then don't buy it. If it isn't in the house you can't eat it during a weak moment. Select other treats instead.

❖ Sometimes it's easier just to skip the aisle with the chocolates, confectionery and biscuits; if this helps you to stay away from temptation then do it!

❖ Go shopping on your own; children and partners can be distracting and can tempt you into buying things you had not planned to purchase.

❖ Look carefully at the labels when you are buying foods and compare brands; go for the lowest-fat options.

❖ Go to the deli counter and buy as much as you need, rather than buying larger packs of pre-packaged foods.

WHAT'S ON A LABEL?

It helps to understand nutrition labelling, as increasingly manufacturers are putting out information to promote their products.

The food label usually lists the nutrients, often given per 100g and per serve, and there may also be nutrition claims. In most countries there are stringent regulations governing the claims that can be made on products.

Most commonly listed in the nutrient information are energy, protein, fat and carbohydrate. There may also be information on saturates, sugars, fibre and sodium.

Some of the terms may be hard to figure out, particularly kilojoules, saturates and carbohydrates. For more information on these terms see Chapter 5. It can also be difficult to apply the information to what you actually need or want on a healthy diet. For example, although most people do wish to reduce their fat intake, very few know exactly how much to consume on a daily basis. The 'guideline daily amounts' for energy, fat and salt, given opposite, should help you to figure out how much you should be consuming. These values apply to a healthy adult who is maintaining his or her weight. The figures in brackets show the reduced amounts required by those on a weight reducing diet.

Guidelines for Energy and Fat Consumption		
	Men	**Women**
Energy (kcal)	2500 (2000)	2000 (1500)
Fat (g)	95 (70)	70 (55)
Salt (g)	7	5

FOOD PREPARATION AND COOKING TIPS

Here are some suggestions for eating healthily when preparing and cooking food.

❖ Don't eat while preparing food.

❖ Don't be afraid to throw away food after the meal. Eating leftovers to save waste, won't save your waist.

❖ If you live alone, prepare meals for four to six and freeze them into individual portions. This is a great way to have healthy 'ready-meals' when you rush in late from work.

❖ Always trim all the visible fat from meat.

❖ Remove and discard the skin from chicken and turkey either before cooking, or before serving.

❖ Buy lean bacon rather than streaky; it may be more expensive but it's best to spend the same amount of money and buy less. You save, as there is less waste.

❖ Try homemade burgers made with lean minced meat as an alternative to shop-bought or takeaway varieties (see Chapter 7 for recipes).

❖ Extend lean meat with pulses (peas, beans, lentils) and lots of vegetables.

❖ Use lower-fat yoghurt, milk and cheese.

❖ Grate cheese rather than slicing – it goes further and you need less.

❖ Dry-fry if possible to avoid adding extra fat to food, or just use a light spray of unsaturated oil.

❖ Grill foods on a rack so excess fat drains away.

❖ Skim fat off the top of casseroles and stews.

❖ Make your own low-fat oven chips or roast potatoes (see Chapter 7 for recipes).

❖ Use skimmed milk rather than butter when mashing vegetables.

❖ Choose lower-fat sauces and salad dressings, and avoid using too much.

❖ Have moist fillings in sandwiches to avoid the need for any fat spreads.

❖ Have dry toast with baked beans; no need for fat spreads here either.

❖ Have a thin scraping of jam on toast instead of butter.

❖ Try serving on smaller plates and bowls to avoid the temptation of serving excessive portions.

PORTION SIZES

One area that causes a lot of confusion is the size of a portion. As food outlets offer increasingly generous servings in order to give good value for money, you can end up with much more than you want or need. It was recently estimated that single combination packages available from well-known fast food outlets provide well in excess of a teenage girl's entire daily energy and fat needs.[1]

We are becoming used to these oversized helpings from a very young age. Research shows that even children as young as five are overeating, rather than stopping when they have had enough.[2] You and your family may need to reassess what constitutes an appropriate serving. As a starting point it may be useful to purchase a set of scales and weigh out standard portions of food, just so you get an idea visually what a portion looks like. Portion sizes for different foods, classified into the different food groups, are given below.

Fruit and Vegetables
Have at least 5 portions per day, and include a variety of types and colours.

2 tblsp raw, cooked, frozen or canned vegetables

Small bowl of salad

1 medium tomato or carrot

1 medium apple, banana, pear or orange

2 medium stone fruit, e.g. apricot or plum

Small bowl of fruit salad (fresh or tinned in natural juice)

1 large slice of melon

½ grapefruit

½ tblsp dried fruit

1 glass (150ml) of fruit juice

Bread, Other Cereals and Potatoes
Choose wholegrain varieties and aim for 5 servings or more a day, depending on your energy needs.

1 medium potato

1 small pitta bread

1 medium slice of bread

2 Weetabix

Small bowl of cornflakes or bran flakes

Small bowl of porridge

Small bowl (2-3 tbsp) of cooked pasta or rice

Milk and Milk Products
Have 3 servings a day and choose the lower fat varieties.

1/3 pint of milk

Small pot of yoghurt

Matchbox-sized piece of cheese

Meat, Fish and Alternatives
Have 2–3 servings a day and trim off all the visible fat.

2 slices cooked meat (e.g. ham or chicken)

1 medium egg

3 tblsp beans or lentils (cooked)

50g-100g (2–4 oz) steak

2 chicken drumsticks

150g (6 oz) fillet of fish

2 tblsp nuts

Foods Containing Fats
Keep these to a minimum.

1 tsp butter, margarine or spread

2 tsp low-fat spread

1 tsp oil

1 small packet of crisps

Foods Containing Sugar
Don't eat these too frequently and limit your intake.

3 tsp sugar

Small (50g/2 oz) bar of chocolate

Small packet (25g/1 oz) sweets/candies

FOOD SWAPS
There are some very simple modifications you can make to cut down on calories and fat. Just by swapping one type of food for a similar alternative you can make a dramatic difference. A few ideas are shown below.

High-calorie/fat Food	Suggested Alternatives	Calorie Saving (kcal)	Fat Saving (g)
Fried cod and fried chips	Grilled cod and oven chips	345	32.0
25g packet of crisps	10g cup of popcorn	85	6.5
Steak and kidney pie	Cottage pie	595	42.0
2 slices of garlic bread	Bread roll	75	9.0
Croissant	Crumpet	105	9.5
Sausage roll	Grilled sausage	150	10.0
100g (4 oz) grilled bacon (with fat)	100g (4 oz) lean ham	230	23.5
1 slice of cheese on toast (Cheddar)	1 slice of cheese on toast (half fat Cheddar)	55	8.0
(Souce: based on data from *McCance and Widdowson's The Composition of Foods*[3])			

To put all this into context, don't forget that an average man who is maintaining his weight on a healthy diet should have around 2500kcal and 95g fat per day; for a woman, the figures are around 2000kcal and 70g fat per day.

For those who are on a weight-reducing plan, calorie intake should be about 2000kcal per day for men and 1500kcal per day for women. Fat intakes should be around 70g and 55g for men and women respectively. These amounts will, of course, vary with differing energy needs and are intended as a rough guide only.

CONVENIENCE FOODS AND FAST FOODS

Most of us couldn't manage without frozen, canned or packaged food. Sometimes these are criticised for being less healthy than fresh food, but there is actually nothing wrong with this option. However, fast foods can be high in fat so be careful where you go and what choices you make; chips, pies and fried foods are all high in fat. Instead choose sandwiches, pizzas with vegetable toppings (but go easy on the cheese), grilled fish or chicken sandwiches, filled jacket potatoes and salads.

Try making your own fast foods at home. It takes only about ten minutes to put together a stir-fry or some delicious low-fat burgers with oven chips (see Chapter 7). This is probably about how long you would spend waiting for your meal in a fast-food outlet or waiting for a takeaway to be delivered.

EATING OUT

When you're in a restaurant, sometimes the best-laid plans can be challenged. Here are a few tips.

❖   Select restaurants and outlets that have healthy options.

❖   Try the sandwich shops that allow you to select your own ingredients.

❖   Stay away from calorie-laden nibbles such as nachos, prawn crackers and poppadoms.

❖   If you really have to take the kids to a burger bar, select a plain burger and ask for it to be prepared specially, with no mayonnaise. Have water, a diet drink, a tea or a coffee to go with it.

❖ At buffet-type restaurants, go for the healthy options and visit the buffet bar only once.

❖ Don't be afraid to ask for information on what's in the different dishes and how they are served. Most restaurants will be happy to modify your meal to suit your needs.

❖ Order a baked potato rather than fries, and extra vegetables or salad to fill you up.

❖ Choose plain rice or noodles rather than fried.

❖ If you are served a giant portion, don't be tempted to eat it all. Ask for the remainder to be packed up for you to take home.

❖ Avoid the temptation to 'super-size' your meal; it may seem like good value but you don't really want or need the extra food, as it will just pile on the weight.

DRINKS
It's important to drink plenty of fluids, especially in hot weather and during heavy exercise, to replace that lost in sweat. The average adult needs at least six to eight cups of fluid a day (1½–2 litres or 3–4 pints).

Water is one of the best options. Try the sparkling mineral waters for a change; add flavours such as lemon juice and mint leaves, or fruit such as oranges and lemons. Top up with ice and serve well chilled in an elegant glass.

Another option for a healthy drink is skimmed milk. Add fruit and low-fat ice cream for a delicious fruit smoothie (see Chapter 7). If you decide to have soft drinks, go for the low-sugar or 'diet' versions.

COMMON MISCONCEPTIONS
There are a lot of myths around when it comes to food; here are a few of the more common ones.

Margarine has fewer calories than butter. FALSE.
All fats, whether they are oils, soft margarines, hard margarines or butter, have the same number of calories. The main difference is in the fatty acids they contain. Butter and hard margarine contain mainly saturated fatty acids, whereas oils and soft margarines contain mainly unsaturated fatty acids (see Chapter 5).

The best option is to go for the low-fat unsaturated spreads, which do actually contain fewer calories.

It's 97 per cent fat-free, so I can eat as much as I like. FALSE.
There is an increasing range of 95–99 per cent fat-free cakes, biscuits and cereal bars, and it's easy to think these are a good option. They are often described as 'guilt-free', giving the impression that you can really indulge and eat as much as you wish. However, they are often high in sugar and calories and not very filling, so it is easy to eat too much.

Before you know it, you'll have eaten a significant number of calories. Instead, try filling up on fruit, vegetables or the treat ideas given in Chapter 7.

Egg yolks are high in cholesterol, so dieters shouldn't eat them. FALSE.
Saturated fatty acids are a more important determinant of blood cholesterol levels than the small amounts of dietary cholesterol found in eggs. Eggs are actually quite a healthy food and can be used in a variety of ways – either incorporated into dishes or poached or boiled and served with dry wholemeal toast. Alternatively, an omelette made with lots of vegetables and served with a large mixed salad makes a nutritious meal. If you enjoy eggs, having up to one a day on average would not pose a problem. Only those with very high cholesterol levels will need to restrict their intake, probably to about two or three eggs a week. People with high cholesterol levels should seek the advice of a dietitian on a diet low in saturated fatty acids and cholesterol.

Honey and brown sugar are better for you than white sugar. FALSE.
Apart from flavour, there really isn't a great deal of difference from a nutritional point of view between the different types of sugar and honey. They are all almost pure carbohydrate, although there is a negligible amount of some minerals in honey. Be careful not to consume too many sugary foods (such as confectionery) and drinks, as these can make a significant contribution to your overall calorie intake if you are not careful.

Red meat is full of fat. FALSE.
Because of the breeds of cattle farmed today, along with modified feeding practices and new butchery techniques, many cuts of red meat are now extremely low in fat. The good thing about meat too is that you can see most of the fat and cut it off. Very lean cuts of pork, such as pork leg steak, are now so low in fat that on a weight-for-weight basis they contain about the same amount of fat as cottage cheese!

Always buy the leanest meat you can afford. Make extra-lean cuts of minced beef go further with dried beans, lentils or vegetables. Try to stay away from meat products (especially those with pastry), which can be high in fat.

Avoid fatty fish when you're on a diet. FALSE.
The omega-3 fatty acids found in fish oils are beneficial to health (see Chapter 5). If you like fish then eat at least one or two portions each week. Salmon, mackerel and sardines are among those that contain the beneficial fatty acids. Serve it steamed, grilled or baked, with lots of delicious fresh herbs, black pepper and lemon juice.

Cocoa is high in fat. FALSE.
One teaspoon of cocoa powder contains less than one gram of fat. If you enjoy chocolate flavours then there is no harm in treating yourself to the odd cup of hot cocoa. Make up the drink using skimmed milk to keep your fat intake low.

Caffeine is bad for you. FALSE.
In fact, caffeine can sometimes be beneficial. If you're feeling a bit tired or run-down, a cup of coffee can really perk you up. Studies have shown that caffeine can help sustain attention during the post-lunch dip, at night, after prolonged work and when a person has a cold. Caffeine is found in coffee, tea, chocolate, cola and cocoa, and in some of the new 'energy drinks' now on the market. Some people are, however, sensitive to caffeine and this can cause them to become irritable or have trouble sleeping. If this applies to you, you may wish to limit your intake of caffeine (particularly in the evening) and find alternative drinks such as decaffeinated coffee or herbal tea. Pregnant women are advised to limit their intake of caffeine to no more than 300mg per day; this is equivalent to about three to four cups of coffee.

Nuts are low in fat. FALSE.
Nuts can be a useful source of nutrients, particularly for vegetarians. However, they can be high in fat (walnuts are 65 per cent fat, and dry-roasted peanuts are 53 per cent) so eat only a small handful rather than a large bowlful, and not too frequently. If you're inclined to nibble on nuts and want a tasty alternative, try the recipes for bread or vegetables with dips in Chapter 7.

7

TIME TO COOK

The aim of this chapter is to dispel the myth that healthy food is boring and unappetising, and to help you develop a positive eating plan based on foods you enjoy. You can eat burgers, chips, pizzas and cakes on the power of positive eating plan; all that's needed are a few modifications to reduce or eliminate the fat content and make sure the portion sizes are correct and the meals are properly balanced with the right proportions of foods from the different food groups. The recipe ideas are really a starting point to give you some ideas on how to prepare foods when aiming to lose weight or eat healthily. Try some of them out for yourself and your family, or try adapting some of your own favourite recipes in a similar way.

We start with a list of equipment that will prove helpful.

EQUIPMENT
Although you don't need any special equipment in order to eat healthily, there are some items that make food preparation, cooking and storage quicker and easier.

Freezer
A freezer is useful as you will be able to prepare bulk meals and freeze them in individual or family-sized portions, saving you time and effort. This is a great, healthy way to enjoy fast food. Foods that can be frozen easily include meat, stews and casseroles, soups and sauces, vegetables and fruit, rice, bread and muffins.

Microwave
A microwave is great for defrosting meals from the freezer and for cooking up meals quickly.

Slow Cooker
Slow cookers, or crock pots, are excellent for cheaper cuts of meat that would be quite tough cooked any other way. Just throw the lean meat, lots of vegetables, a couple of stock cubes and a tin of tomatoes into the cooker in the morning, then turn it on and forget about it until dinnertime. With a little planning, a slow cooker helps to take the stress out of a busy day as you come home to a delicious meal.

Rice Cooker
Steamed rice is a delicious accompaniment to any meal, and with a rice cooker you can make it to perfection. Just place the rice and water in the cooker, turn it on and it will do everything for you. With some models you can steam vegetables over the rice at the same time.

Hand Blender
A hand-held blender is ideal for making soups, sauces, fruit smoothies and fruit juices with blended fruit. This is a relatively inexpensive investment.

Yoghurt Maker
In the long run, yoghurt can be a lot cheaper if you make your own. There are various low-fat flavours and it's easy to make. Low-fat yoghurt is a great snack, dessert or accompaniment for fresh fruit.

Wok
You can cook almost anything in a wok, but they are especially good for Chinese-style stir-fries. Choose a non-stick type, to avoid the need for too much oil. Spray lightly with an unsaturated oil and fry lean meats with lots of vegetables. Serve with potatoes, rice, pasta or pitta bread for a quick, easy, healthy meal.

Baking Tray
A quality non-stick baking tray is a worthwhile investment to aid fat-free cooking. You could also use non-stick paper to line a baking tray.

Wire Rack
Invest in a wire rack that will allow the fat to run off your food. This will come in useful for both grilling and roasting meat and other foods.

HYGIENE TIPS
Good hygiene practices when preparing, cooking, storing and reheating foods will help to ensure your food is wholesome and fit to eat. Key points to remember are shown below.

❖   Always wash your hands thoroughly before preparing food, and cover any cuts and grazes.

❖   Keep chopping boards and equipment for raw and cooked food separate.

❖   Keep waste bins covered and away from food.

❖   Keep pets away from the kitchen.

❖   Wash thoroughly all food to be eaten raw.

❖   Thaw frozen meat completely before cooking.

❖   Cook meat to an internal temperature of at least 75°C (167°F).

❖   When cooking meat products such as burgers or sausages, ensure they are cooked through until the juices run clear and no pink bits remain.

❖   Cool food quickly and refrigerate, particularly meat, fish and eggs.

❖   Cover all food before storage.

❖ Make sure the fridge is running at a temperature of less than 4°C (39°F) and the freezer less than –18°C (0°F).

❖ Do not overload the fridge or leave the door open for longer than necessary.

❖ Cover all foods and keep raw meat at the bottom of the fridge to avoid juices dripping onto other food.

❖ Store eggs in the fridge.

❖ Always use food by the expiry of the use-by date.

❖ Reheat food thoroughly until it is piping hot. Never reheat more than once.

MEAL PLANS

It isn't a good idea to follow rigid, pre-set meal plans because they are so hard to stick to. However, having a rough idea of the types of foods to eat and the number of portions to include at each meal can be a useful starting point in re-educating your eating habits.

Page 94 contains a meal plan for weight loss; page 95 a meal plan for healthy eating/weight maintenance. Remember these are just a rough guide. A manual worker who is 6 ft (1.83m) tall will need a much higher energy intake than an office worker who is 5 ft (1.52m). Adjust the plans to suit your own needs, depending on the rate of weight-loss you are aiming for. If, for example, you cook a stir-fry, you may wish to mix together in a wok two portions of rice or noodles, one portion of lean meat and two portions of vegetables. For information on portion sizes, see Chapter 6.

Don't forget that meals don't need to be the traditional 'meat and veg' formula; a mix-and-match approach is perfectly all right as well.

RECIPE IDEAS

Pages 96–116 contain a selection of recipe ideas that are designed to be quick and easy to prepare. The different ideas are divided into:

- ❖ Main meals: pages 96–101.
- ❖ Accompaniments: pages 102–104.
- ❖ Light meals: pages 105–110.
- ❖ Dips: page 111.
- ❖ Desserts: pages 112–113.
- ❖ Treats: pages 114–116.

	Weight-loss Meal Plan
Breakfast	1 portion of wholegrain breakfast cereal with ½ pint of skimmed or semi-skimmed milk *or* 1–2 slices of toast with a scraping of low-fat spread and/or jam 1 portion of fruit
Mid-morning	Small wholemeal scone or a low-fat muffin *or* piece of fruit
Lunch	1–2 portions of bread Scraping of low-fat spread 1 portion of lean meat, poultry, beans, egg or low-fat cheese Large mixed salad Low-fat yoghurt Piece of fruit
Mid-afternoon	Piece of fruit
Dinner	1 portion of lean meat, fish or beans 1–2 portions of rice, pasta, noodles or potatoes 2–3 portions of vegetables Fresh fruit salad
Supper	2 plain crackers or crispbreads with low-fat cheese *or* 1 slice of toast with a scraping of low-fat spread and/or jam

	Weight-maintenance Meal Plan
Breakfast	1 portion of wholegrain breakfast cereal with $\frac{1}{2}$ pint of skimmed or semi-skimmed milk
	1–2 slices of toast with a scraping of margarine or low-fat spread and/or jam
	1 portion of fruit
Mid-morning	Wholemeal scone, muffin or piece of fruit cake
	Piece of fruit
Lunch	2 portions of bread
	Scraping of margarine or low-fat spread
	1 portion of lean meat, poultry, beans, egg or low-fat cheese
	Large mixed salad
	Low-fat yoghurt
	Piece of fruit
Mid-afternoon	Wholemeal scone, muffin or piece of fruit cake
	Piece of fruit
Dinner	1 portion of lean meat, fish or beans
	2–3 portions of rice, pasta, noodles or potatoes
	2–3 portions of vegetables
	Fresh fruit salad
Supper	2 plain crackers or crispbreads with low-fat cheese
	or 1–2 slices of toast with a scraping of margarine or low-fat spread and/or jam

MAIN MEALS

Meat Casserole (serves 4–6)

Ingredients
400g (1 lb) lean trimmed beef, lamb or pork, or skinless
  chicken fillets
2 medium onions, peeled and chopped
3 carrots, peeled and chopped
3 parsnips, peeled and chopped
250g (10 oz) mushrooms, washed and chopped
1 large (400g) tin tomatoes
1 packet casserole mix (or a selection of herbs and 2 stock
  cubes)

Method
1. Spray a frying pan or wok lightly with oil.
2. Fry the meat until browned.
3. Add the onions and sauté the meat and onions
   together for 5 mins.
4. Add the carrots, parsnips and mushrooms. Cook for
   a further 5 mins.
5. Add the tomatoes and the casserole mix (or herbs
   and stock cubes). Cook for a further 5 mins.
6. Pour the mixture into a casserole dish. Bake at 180°C/
   350°F/gas mark 4 for 1½ hours.

Serve with vegetables and potatoes.

Tips
❖ For fresh, close-to-hand flavours, grow some herbs
   such as parsley, chives and basil on your kitchen
   window sill.
❖ A good alternative to meat for vegetarians is mixed
   beans and pulses.
❖ This type of meal works well in a slow cooker if you
   want to go for the cheaper cuts of meat.

Cheesy Crunchy Vegetable Bake (serves 4–6)

Ingredients
3 medium carrots
1 medium onion
25g (1 oz) mushrooms
1 bunch celery
1 packet cheese sauce mix
2 tbsp grated low-fat cheese
2 tbsp breadcrumbs

Method
1.   Peel the carrots and chop into batons.
2.   Peel and chop the onion.
3.   Slice the mushrooms.
4.   Lightly spray a non-stick frying pan or wok with oil.
5.   Sauté the carrots, onion and mushrooms for approximately 10 mins on a low heat.
6.   Meanwhile wash and chop the celery.
7.   Boil the celery for 5 mins.
8.   Drain the celery and stir into the vegetable mixture.
9.   Place all the vegetables into a casserole dish and bake for 40 mins at 200°C/400°F/gas mark 6.
10. Prepare the cheese sauce according to the instructions on the packet.
11. Pour over the vegetable mix.
12. Sprinkle over the grated cheese and breadcrumbs.
13. Bake for a further 20 mins.

Serve with rice, pasta, potatoes or pitta bread.

ли Con Carne (serves 4–6)

Ingredients
2 medium onions, chopped
400g (1 lb) extra lean minced beef
1 large (420g) tin kidney beans
1 large (400g) tin tomatoes
1 packet dried chilli mix

Method
1. Lightly spray a large frying pan or wok with oil.
2. Fry the onions on a low heat for 5 mins until soft.
3. Add the meat and fry until thoroughly browned.
4. Drain the kidney beans and stir into the meat mixture.
5. Stir in the tomatoes.
6. Add the dried chilli mix, cook over a low heat for a further 5 mins.
7. Place the chilli in a large casserole dish and bake at 180°C/350°F/gas mark 4 for 1 hour.

Serve with rice.

Spaghetti Bolognese (serves 4–6)

Ingredients
2 medium onions, chopped
400g (1 lb) extra lean minced beef
1 large (400g) tin tomatoes
1 packet of dried bolognese mix
1 tsp mixed dried herbs

Method
1. Lightly spray a large frying pan or wok with oil.
2. Fry the onions on a low heat for 5 mins until soft.
3. Add the meat and fry until thoroughly browned.

4. Stir in the tomatoes.
5. Add the dried bolognese mix and herbs, cook over a low heat for a further 5 mins.
6. Place the bolognese in a large casserole dish and bake at 180°C/350°F/gas mark 4 for 1 hour.

Serve with spaghetti, warmed French bread and a side salad.

Chow Mein (serves 4–6)

Ingredients
1 packet (400g) noodles
1 medium onion
100g (4 oz) mushrooms
2 medium green peppers
2 chilli peppers (be careful to wash your hands straight after handling the chillies as they can sting)
400g (1 lb) lean trimmed beef, lamb or pork, or skinless chicken fillets
soy sauce to season

Method
1. Place the noodles in a pan and add boiling water.
2. Boil for 2 mins until soft.
3. Drain.
4. Meanwhile, lightly spray a large frying pan or wok with oil.
5. Chop the vegetables and fry gently over a low heat for 5 mins.
6. Chop the meat finely and add to the vegetables.
7. Continue to cook over a low heat until the meat is cooked – about 10 mins.
8. Add the noodles.
9. Cook for a further 5 mins.
10. Season with soy sauce.

Serve with a mixed salad.

Delicious Vegetable Pasta Bake (serves 4–6)

Ingredients
400g (1 lb) pasta
1 medium onion
1 medium green pepper
100g (4 oz) mushrooms
1 portion salsa sauce (see recipe on page 111) or 1 jar
  (400g) pasta sauce
100g (4 oz) lean ham, chopped (optional)
50g (2 oz) low-fat cheese, grated
1 tsp dried mixed herbs
pinch salt and pepper

Method
1. Place the pasta in a large saucepan and cover with boiling water.
2. Simmer for 8–10 mins, or until the pasta is *al dente* (firm).
3. Drain. Place pasta in a large casserole dish.
4. Chop the vegetables.
5. Lightly spray a frying pan or wok with oil and fry the vegetables over a low heat for 5 mins.
6. Add the vegetables to the pasta.
7. Stir in the sauce.
8. Sprinkle over chopped ham if desired.
9. Top with grated cheese and herbs.
10. Season with salt and pepper.
11. Microwave on high for 5 mins in a 750 watt microwave (note you may need to adjust the cooking time depending on your microwave). Or bake at 180°C/ 350°F/gas mark 4 for 20 mins.

Serve with a crisp green salad and a small toasted pitta bread.

Burgers (serves 4–6)

Ingredients
400g (1 lb) extra lean minced beef
salt and pepper to taste
1 tsp dried mixed herbs
4–6 bread rolls
tomato or chilli sauce
vegetables (shredded lettuce, sliced tomato, chopped
 onion, peppers)
4–6 thin slices low-fat cheese (optional)

Method
1. Mix the mince with the salt, pepper and herbs in a
    bowl.
2. Divide into four to six portions.
3. Roll each portion into a ball, then flatten into a
    circular shape.
4. Grill until cooked thoroughly all the way through –
    about 10 mins.

To serve
1. Slice in half a bread roll for each burger and toast on
    one side only.
2. Place the burger on the roll, add tomato or chilli
    sauce and vegetables. As a treat, add a thin slice of
    low-fat cheese.
3. Serve with one portion of low-fat oven chips (see
    recipe on page 103, or try the frozen variety that has
    less than 5 per cent fat).

ACCOMPANIMENTS

Boiled Rice (serves 2–4)
1. Place 150g (6 oz) rice in a saucepan.
2. Add 340ml (12 fl oz) boiling water.
3. Cover and simmer for 15–20 mins.
4. Serve.

Microwaved Rice (serves 2–4)
1. Place 150g (6 oz) rice in a non-metallic bowl.
2. Add 340ml (12 fl oz) boiling water.
3. Microwave for 18 mins on high power in a 750 watt microwave (note: you may need to adjust the cooking time depending on your microwave).
4. Serve.

Tips
❖ Don't worry about cooking too much rice, as it freezes well and can be reheated in the microwave.
❖ Use as a base for salads, add to stir-fries, or simply serve with the main meal.

Boiled Potatoes
1. Peel one medium potato per person, chop into cubes and place in a saucepan.
2. Cover with boiling water.
3. Boil for approximately 10 mins.
4. Drain and serve as they are or mash with skimmed milk and seasoning.

Jacket Potatoes
1. Wash and prick potatoes.
2. Microwave on high in a 750 watt microwave for 4 mins (see note above) per medium-sized potato.

Roast/Chipped Potatoes

1. Peel potatoes and cut into chips (or quarters, for roast potatoes).
2. Microwave on high in a 750 watt microwave for 3 mins (see note opposite) per medium-sized potato, or parboil.
3. Place on a baking tray covered with silicon paper.
4. Spray lightly with oil.
5. Bake for 20–30 mins at 180°C/350°F/gas mark 4.

Tips

❖ Potatoes can form the basis of a snack or salad, or accompany the main meal.

❖ Be careful not to add fat to jacket or mashed potatoes.

❖ As a topping for jacket potatoes try wholegrain mustard, chilli sauce, chutney, low-fat yoghurt or fromage frais.

❖ Try sweet potatoes or other root vegetables as a delicious alternative.

Pasta (serves 4–6)

1. Place 400g (1 lb) pasta in a saucepan.
2. Cover with boiling water and bring back to the boil.
3. Simmer for 8–10 mins, or until the pasta is *al dente* (firm).
4. Drain and serve.

Tips

❖ Buy different-shaped or coloured pasta for variety.
❖ Try it as a basis for salads.

Breads

Bread is a great accompaniment to a meal and there is a huge variety in supermarkets and shops. Try toasting pitta bread straight from the freezer, or try breads that are baked with herbs, onions, tomatoes and other delicious flavours. Choose plenty of different types to keep your food interesting and enjoyable.

Salad

In the summer, keep plenty of your favourite salad vegetables in the fridge. These can be great on sandwiches, and with light or main meals. Be careful not to use high-fat salad dressings; just a little lemon juice and black pepper can make a tasty dressing.

Prepared salads save time but can be expensive. It's cheaper to buy the vegetables, wash them, chop them and refrigerate them in a big salad container. Use lettuce, beans, tomatoes, beetroot, cucumber, cress, carrots, onions, peppers, radishes. You could also add fruit such as oranges, strawberries, pineapple and kiwi fruit.

Vegetables

Don't forget to include fresh vegetables on your shopping list each week. Go for the ones that are in season as these are usually cheaper. Pre-prepared vegetables are becoming more widely available, but like salads are often very expensive.

Always have a ready supply of frozen vegetables too – either shop-bought or home frozen – for boiling, microwaving or steaming.

LIGHT MEALS

Tomato Soup (serves 2)

Ingredients
6 medium tomatoes
1 tsp dried mixed herbs
1 fresh chilli (be careful to wash your hands straight after
   handling chillies as they can sting)

Method
1. Place the tomatoes in a covered dish and microwave
    for 5 mins in a 750 watt microwave (note: you may
    need to adjust the cooking time depending on your
    microwave).
2. Using a hand blender or liquidiser purée the toma-
    toes.
3. Add the herbs and chopped chilli.
4. Microwave for 1 min on high, or boil in a saucepan.

Serve with dry bread or toast.

Tip
❖   Use a large tin of tomatoes as a quick alternative.

Potato Soup (serves 4)

Ingredients
4 medium-sized potatoes, peeled and diced
1 onion, peeled and chopped
2 vegetable stock cubes
250ml ($\frac{1}{2}$ pint) skimmed milk
$\frac{1}{2}$ tsp basil
pinch salt and pepper
1 tsp coriander
1 tsp cumin
1 tsp turmeric

Method
1. Place the potatoes and onions in a saucepan and add 750ml ($1\frac{1}{2}$ pints) water.
2. Bring to the boil and simmer for about 10–15 mins until cooked.
3. Add the remaining ingredients.
4. Purée using a hand blender or liquidiser.

Serve with dry bread or toast.

Parsnip Soup (serves 4)

Ingredients
1 medium onion
6 medium parsnips
250ml (½ pint) skimmed milk
½ banana
1 tsp curry powder
1 tsp turmeric
pinch salt and pepper

Method
1. Peel and chop the onion.
2. Peel and chop the parsnips.
3. Place the vegetables in a large saucepan and cover with 750ml (1½ pints) of boiling water.
4. Bring to the boil, then simmer for approximately 10–15 mins until the vegetables are soft.
5. Add the milk and banana.
6. Purée using a hand blender or liquidiser.
7. Add the curry powder and turmeric, and salt and pepper to taste.

Serve with dry bread or toast.

Tips
❖   Soup freezes well, and is ideal for lunch at home or at work.
❖   Buy packet or canned soups and stir in some extra vegetables.

Pizza (serves 2)

Ingredients
bread base (1 French stick, or 2 pitta breads, or 2 shop-
    bought pizza bases approximately 12cm (5 in) in dia-
    meter)
150g (5 oz) tomato paste/purée
200g (8 oz) creamed sweetcorn (or purée 1 can standard
    sweetcorn)
2 tbsp low-fat grated cheese
10g (½ oz) lean ham, chopped (optional)
2 tbsp vegetables (onions, mushrooms, peppers, tomatoes)

Method
1. If using a French stick, slice in half to make two
    bases.
2. Spread half the tomato purée over each base.
3. Top with half the creamed corn.
4. Sprinkle with 1 tbsp grated cheese.
5. Add chopped ham (if desired) and mixed vegetables.
6. Bake for 10 mins at 200°C/400°F/gas mark 6.

Serve with a crisp green salad.

Cheesy Bean Baskets (serves 2–3)

Ingredients
6 thick slices bread
1 large (420g) tin baked beans
3 tbsp low-fat grated cheese
25g (1 oz) lean ham (optional)

Method
1. Lightly grease a large six-muffin tray.
2. Place a saucer over each slice of bread and cut around it to remove the crusts, leaving a circular piece.
3. Mould the bread into the muffin tray.
4. Bake for 10 mins at 200°C/400°F/gas mark 6.
5. Heat the beans in a microwave or a saucepan.
6. Fill each bread basket with beans.
7. Top each with ¹/₂ tbsp grated cheese.
8. Sprinkle with 1 tsp ham if desired.
9. Return to the oven for 5 mins.

Tip
❖   As an alternative to beans try spaghetti in tomato sauce.

Jacket Potatoes with Cheese and Beans (serves 2)

Ingredients
2 medium-sized potatoes
1 large (420g) tin baked beans
2 tbsp low-fat grated cheese

Method
1. Wash and prick the potatoes and microwave for 8–10 mins in a 750 watt microwave (note: you may need to adjust the cooking time depending on your micro-wave).
2. Slice the potatoes in half.
3. Pour over baked beans (preheated in the microwave or heated on the stove).
4. Top with grated cheese.

DIPS

Salsa

Ingredients
1 large (400g) tin tomatoes
1 green pepper, chopped
1 onion, chopped
2–3 chilli peppers, chopped (be careful to wash your hands straight after handling chillies as they sting)

Method
1. Put all the ingredients in a bowl.
2. Blend with a hand blender or liquidiser.

Yoghurt Dip

Ingredients
sprig fresh mint leaves
125g pot low-fat plain yoghurt
50g (2 oz) cucumber

Method
1. Chop the mint leaves.
2. Stir into the yoghurt.
3. Finely dice cucumber and add to the yoghurt.

Tip
❖ Serve dips with a selection of breads or chopped vegetables (e.g. carrots, celery, peppers, broccoli, courgettes, cauliflower).

DESSERTS

Crunchy Apple Crumble (serves 6)

Ingredients
8 eating apples, unpeeled, cored and cut into quarters
1 tsp mixed spice
50g (2 oz) low-fat spread
60g (2½ oz) plain flour
50g (2 oz) rolled oats
100g (4 oz) demerara sugar

Method
1. Chop the apples in a food processor, or grate by hand.
2. Put the fruit straight into a pudding bowl and combine with the mixed spice.
3. To make the crumble topping, rub the low-fat spread into the flour. Stir in the oats and sugar.
4. Sprinkle the crumble topping over the fruit.
5. Bake for 20 mins at 180°C/350°F/gas mark 4.

Tips
❖ Use a deep bowl with a small diameter to get maximum fruit.
❖ Try different types of fruit – fresh, canned or frozen.
❖ Serve with low-fat ice cream, yoghurt, or custard made with skimmed milk.

Pavlova (serves 4–6)

Ingredients
4 medium egg whites
100g (4 oz) caster sugar
100g (4 oz) topping: cold custard, yoghurt, low-fat fromage frais or low-fat ice cream
400g tinned or fresh fruit (oranges, pineapple, berry fruit
or kiwi fruit)

Method
1. Whisk up the egg whites until firm.
2. Fold in the caster sugar.
3. Pile the meringue mixture onto a baking tray covered
    with non-stick paper.
4. Bake at 150°C/300°F/gas mark 2 for 45 mins.
5. Leave to cool.
6. Serve with your choice of topping.
7. Decorate with lots of your favourite fruit.

Tuttifrutti Ice Cream (serves 1)

Ingredients
2 tbsp low-fat ice cream
2 tbsp fresh, tinned or frozen berry fruit

Method
1. Place ingredients in a jug.
2. Mix together with a hand blender.

TREATS

Gooey Sultana Muffins (makes 24 mini-muffins)

Ingredients
125ml (¼ pint) skimmed milk
1 egg
125g (5 oz) self-raising flour
100g (4 oz) oats
100g (4 oz) soft brown sugar
75g (3 oz) sultanas
6 tsp jam (any flavour)

Method
1. Mix the milk and egg with a fork.
2. In a separate bowl stir together the flour, oats, sugar and sultanas.
3. Make a well in the centre of the dry ingredients and stir in the milk and egg.
4. Mix together lightly, don't overmix.
5. Lightly spray a mini-muffin tray with oil.
6. Half-fill the tray with mixture, add ¼ tsp jam to each muffin and top with the remaining mixture.
7. Bake at 180°C/350°F/gas mark 4 for 10–15 mins.

Tips
❖ Remember two muffins of this size make one portion.
❖ Freeze muffins and take out one or two each day for morning tea.
❖ If you don't have a muffin tray, use paper cases.

Currant Tea Bread (serves 10)

Ingredients
175g (6 oz) currants
125ml (¼ pint) tea
4 tbsp (100g/4 oz) honey
1 egg
200g (8 oz) self-raising flour
25g (1 oz) melted butter

Method
1. Put the currants, tea and honey in a bowl. Leave to soak for 1 hour.
2. Stir in the egg, flour and melted butter.
3. Pour the mixture into a greased loaf tin.
4. Bake for 35 mins at 180°C/350°F/gas mark 4.
5. Cool and slice.
6. Store in an airtight container.

Fruit Juice Drink (serves 1)

1. Pour 200ml (8 fl oz) fruit juice into a jug.
2. Add a handful of your favourite fruit.
3. Blend with a hand blender or liquidiser.

Tips

❖ Try canned or fresh peaches, pears, or pineapples.
❖ This is a great way of getting fussy children to eat extra fruit.

Fruit Smoothie (serves 1)

1. Place 200ml (8 fl oz) skimmed milk in a jug.
2. Add 2 tbsp low-fat ice cream.
3. Add a handful of your favourite fruit (fresh, frozen or canned).
4. Blend using a hand blender or liquidiser.

Tips

❖ Berry fruits work particularly well.
❖ As an alternative to ice cream try low-fat frozen yoghurt.

8

LET'S TALK PHYSICAL

Our ancestors had much more activity in their lives than we have today. They would have a multitude of daily chores such as washing the clothes by hand, milking the cows and churning the butter. They often cycled or walked to work and had professions that required physical activity, and this meant their level of energy expenditure was significant. In today's society, we have changed the way we live with inventions such as cars, computers and dishwashers, along with a whole range of other labour-saving devices. Also, with the advent of computer technology, many more people work in sedentary jobs. We have remote controls for just about everything in the house these days so we don't even have to get out of our comfy armchairs to change channels on the television or to turn up the volume of the CD player. All these factors have contributed to a lifestyle where we continually have to be creative in how we will burn energy. Our bodies are designed to be active, and the inactivity of today's culture can be viewed as an abnormal state that we need to reverse to avoid ill health and to achieve optimal functioning.

ACTIVITY LEVELS
Your extra weight is made up of fat stores. The processes involved in gaining extra fat are extremely complex. However, one thing is certain: excess weight can only be gained when energy intake (what we eat) remains higher than energy expenditure (our activity), over an extended period

of time. This is influenced by our biology, by our behaviour and by our environment. The key is to look not only at what we are eating but also at how active we are; and to lose weight, we need to expend more energy than we take in.

THE RISKS OF INACTIVITY

Physical inactivity has been described as the fourth major risk factor for heart disease after smoking, high blood fats and high blood pressure.[1] It can also put you at greater risk of other illnesses, and being inactive can mean that you are twice as likely to die younger.[2] So there's plenty of incentive to start moving. But remember, always seek medical advice before undertaking any exercise programme if you have a pre-existing medical condition.

GETTING STARTED

Often, people worry about getting started with exercise, believing it will involve a major commitment in terms of time and energy. People are often relieved to find that just increasing activities such as walking and gardening could benefit them immensely. For these kinds of activities you wouldn't even need to change into any exercise gear, spend any money or involve anyone else.

THE BENEFITS OF EXERCISE

Not only does exercising and keeping fit reduce your health risks; as shown below, it also brings a wide range of other benefits.

- ❖ Helps in weight control.
- ❖ Reduces risk of high blood pressure.
- ❖ Aids management of adult-onset diabetes.
- ❖ Improves functional capacity.
- ❖ Favourably modifies blood fats.

❖   Reduces depression and anxiety.

❖   Improves self-esteem and well-being.

❖   Raises energy levels.

❖   Improves sleep.

❖   Helps to manage stress.

❖   Aids mental relaxation.

❖   Gives you a break from other areas of your life.

❖   Makes you feel great.

As noted above, another great thing about exercise is that it is a good antidote to feelings of depression and anxiety. This is because it stimulates the production of 'feel-good' chemicals in the body.

WHAT DOES EXERCISE MEAN TO YOU?
Perhaps it's doing some boring activity with skimpy clothing on with people laughing at you as you are gasping for breath. It doesn't have to be like that. What you need to decide upon is what is the best type of activity for you. Work out what doesn't cause you to feel embarrassed or uncomfortable, how much time you have, and the added bonus is that you may find it fun.

WHY YOU ARE GOING TO MAKE IT HAPPEN FOR YOU
What will keep you in the ball game? This is different for each of us. Take a few minutes to work out your motivation. It's time to get off that 'on again off again' cycle. Pick up a pen and write down why you want this for you, and have a look at the list overleaf for suggestions on ways to motivate yourself. Is it just the fact that you know that it will develop the body you want to take through this life? Is it to keep a medical condition in check? Take a few minutes to work out the reasons why you want to get fitter.

❖   Preventing a medical condition.

❖   Keeping a medical condition in check.

❖   Keeping up with the children as they play games or run in the park.

❖   Having the energy for sex with your partner after a busy day.

❖   Wanting to be fit for an enjoyable activity or sport.

❖   Being fit for your job.

❖   To look and feel healthier.

❖   To tone your body.

❖   To live longer.

❖   To feel fitter and more energetic.

❖   To shed a few pounds.

❖   To make new friends.

❖   To have fun.

It might be that you can get motivated by meeting new people and getting involved in group exercise schemes. It is likely that with support from our peers we will achieve a much better rate of success.

CHILDREN AND WEIGHT

Encourage your kids to get active, and start by setting an example. Children of inactive parents can pick up bad habits, so as a parent you will feel a responsibility to get more exercise. We certainly don't want to add excess weight to our children's burdens in life.

Letting our children sit in front of the television and computer all day will only pass on the couch-potato lifestyle to the next generation. Think about family activities that are fun – a game of cricket or beach volleyball, or packing up a picnic and going on a bike ride or a long walk, or going to the local swimming pool. Think about what you and your children will enjoy and instigate this into your regular routine.

TYPES OF MOVEMENT
When you start to design your exercise plan, just remember that any movement expends energy, but it is particularly useful to partake in movement that involves larger muscle groups and that involves moving uphill either on a slope or up stairs. It has been suggested[3] that those of us who are overweight should:

❖ Include more weight-bearing movement as part of our daily lives, for example walk up some or all of the stairs instead of taking a lift; make several trips a day up a sloped drive or a nearby road.

❖ Spend less time in sedentary pursuits such as watching television and gradually make activity part of our daily lifestyle, for example through gardening, walking the dog, walking to the shops or washing the car.

❖ Build up to bouts of gentle exercise sustained for 40 minutes or more at a time.

Even though lower-intensity activities burn less energy than more vigorous types of activity, it is likely to occur more frequently, be more sustainable and amount to a significant amount of energy expenditure over a period of weeks, months and years, and that's what we are aiming for. The ultimate aim is both to increase daily activity and to incorporate extended periods of moderate to vigorous activity into our regular routine.

DON'T PUT OFF UNTIL TOMORROW WHAT YOU CAN DO TODAY!
It's all too easy to put off getting started until tomorrow but there's no time like the present to get started on your new life.

Even if you do just one action today you will have made progress; be it to ring a local gym or activity group, tell a friend, or maybe even actually to do some exercise or activity.

If you can find an activity that you enjoy, that you find to be fun, that is fantastic. The truth is that for some of us exercise is not our first choice of activity. It may take time to change the way you feel about exercise but it is something you have to achieve in order to have the health and vitality to live the life you want. There may be a little trial and error involved in finding an activity that you enjoy; enjoyment is important in order to sustain the activity and is the number one factor in identifying what will work for you.

WHAT'S BEST FOR YOU?

Once you have decided to get going, the next stage is to think about what type of person you are. Are you a loner, or a social animal? Are you easily embarrassed, or do you not care what other people think? Do you love buying the latest exercise gear, or would you rather just wear what's in the wardrobe? There may be a little trial and error in finding an activity that you like, but it must be enjoyable if you are to stick with it.

It may be an exercise video or book that enables you to get active in the privacy of your home, or it may be a walk in the neighbourhood, a trip to the local swimming pool, a visit to the gym, or joining a local club. If the first one doesn't feel right, try something else, and you will soon find something that suits you.

Make it Sociable

Can you mix some physical activity into your social life? There are many ways in which you can get active and meet people at the same time. Dancing is a good example – ballroom, ceroc, Latin American, line or even just boogie-ing at the local disco! Or you could join a sports team at work to play badminton, tennis or even indoor netball or cricket.

Be a Copycat

Re-evaluate how you look at people who exercise. Note how they make it happen in their lives, and use it as an example. Some of your work colleagues may run every lunchtime, or do an aerobics class. A determining factor for this may be whether you have access to a shower at work. Talk to your friends and relatives, and see whether you can go along to their local club or gym; people are often happy to show you the ropes if you just ask.

Partner up

Find someone with a positive attitude who is at a similar level, who can exercise with you or support you. Arrange for your new 'exercise buddy' to phone or email you to give support; you can do the same for him or her. Having someone to get active with is a great motivating factor. When you come home feeling tired and thinking it would be easier just to turn on the television, there is always the thought that you can't let your friend down if you've arranged to go for a walk.

Reward Effort

It's all too easy to reward yourself with food, thinking you have done some exercise and now deserve an enormous piece of chocolate cake with whipped cream! Of course, the odd treats are fine, but don't use the fact that you are now in a regular exercise routine as an excuse to overeat on all those fatty and sugary foods. The idea of rewards other than food may be a rather foreign concept, but think about how you can treat yourself in ways that don't involve food. Buy yourself a piggy bank and put some money in it every time you exercise. Use the money to treat yourself to a new book or magazine or even a manicure or facial.

Keep Positive

Don't wait for others to praise you. Tell yourself every day how well you are doing. It's so easy to believe our mind chatter when it says we should be doing better, comparing ourselves to someone else. Be kind to yourself and don't set goals that are too ambitious as you'll just set yourself up for failure and end up disappointed and frustrated. You need to do what's right for you right now. Take things one minute, then one day, then one week, then one month, then one year at a time.

ATTITUDES TO EXERCISE

Become conscious of what you think and say about exercise. Are you saying, 'This is too hard', or, 'I'm too tired'? Change it into a positive, such as, 'This will get easier every day', or 'It's hard to believe, but afterwards I always feel great.' Note what you say and think about other people who are exercising. Are you being negative? Rather than thinking, 'I resent her because she is so fit and happy', tell yourself, 'She's doing really well – I aspire to being like her.' By changing your thought patterns in this way you will create a really powerful position rather than being a victim or a cynic. The following table shows some examples of how to trick the brain into positives.

Negative Thoughts	Positive Thoughts
I don't have the strength to change how I am.	I am a powerful person.
I'm not going to the pool – someone might see me.	There are people of all shapes and sizes at the pool. I'll just go and enjoy myself.
Gyms are just for the young and beautiful.	Gyms are for everybody.
I really don't have the time.	I can make time by getting well organised.

Negative Thoughts	Positive Thoughts
I'm a mother, not a gym instructor.	I am an excellent and fit mother. I can do anything I want with my life.
I have no energy at the end of the day.	Being fitter will make me feel more energetic.
Jogging and walking are so boring.	Jogging and walking are fun.
I tried it once and gave up.	I just need to build up very slowly.
I couldn't afford the gym membership.	Lots of types of exercise are free. I'll get into a walking programme to start with.
I'll injure myself.	I'll manage injuries if I need to.
I've just done a full day at work, fed the children and now I'm exhausted.	A bit of activity will be invigorating and give me some time to myself.

MOTIVATION IS FLAGGING

If once you have started on an exercise regimen you feel you are losing your motivation, assess where you are at the current time. Take some time to think about where you are at in a larger sense. Are you reacting to the boss who wants you to work through a lunch hour when you had organised to do some exercise? Have you overcommitted your time in other areas? Did a friend ring when you were just about to exercise and did you make them more important than yourself? Of course, there is a balance but if you are dropping in your motivation maybe you have made these things more important as an excuse not to exercise. We are all so busy and can easily find other things to do to fill our time. Making time for exercise is a major commitment and you do need to keep motivated to sustain any activity. If you have wandered off the activity and exercise path, start back slowly and don't expect to be at the same level you were at a week or so ago. Also, take comfort that your fitness will bounce back quicker than you expect. Be prepared to get back on that bike when you fall off; don't give in.

Using Variety
If you are a creature of habit and do not get bored with one particular exercise then stay with it. But if you find you are reducing what you are doing, consider putting some variety into your day because it keeps the adventure and spice in ordinary daily activities. The list below gives some ideas to keep things interesting on the activity front.

❖   Change something about the activity.

❖   Exercise at a different time of day.

❖   Walk the other way round the block.

❖   Wear something different.

❖   Combine it with another activity like meditating at the beach or reading by the river.

❖   Talk to the person next to you.

❖   Laugh.

❖   Share your difficulties with friends – they can be a great source of inspiration and ideas.

MISCONCEPTIONS AND EXCUSES
Now let's take a look at some of the misconceptions we hold and excuses we make about exercise.

Spot-reducing
Spot-reducing means slimming down just one part of the body. Some so-called experts will say, for example, that you can reduce the size of your tummy or your thighs by

doing abdominal or thigh exercises. Exercising specific muscles does shorten and strengthen (tone) the muscles in that area, and will hold you a little firmer, but it will not reduce the fat tissue on top of the tummy or around your thighs. Getting the energy balance right is the only way to reduce the amount of fat in your body.

Cellulite
Cellulite is nothing more than a trendy name for fat that is slightly dimpled. You will see magical cures, from diets and passive exercise to creams, lotions, baths and massages. Unfortunately there is no specific cure for cellulite, but by sensible dieting and regular exercise you will reduce the amount of fat in your body, including the dimpled variety.

No Pain, no Gain
You don't have to suffer in order to benefit from exercise, and this is not what we are suggesting here. Although you may not get it right first time, and find that you have muscles that you never knew existed, on the whole if you are in pain then you are not working at an appropriate level. Initially, moderate exercise for sustained periods each day is the key.

I'm short of breath and sweating – this can't be good for me
Being short of breath and sweating is a natural response to 'huff and puff' aerobic exercise. Maintain a level where you can hold a conversation while exercising. If, however, you have any of the conditions listed at the beginning of Chapter 9, seek your doctor's advice.

I'm not doing that – I've never done it before
Are you so set in your ways that you're not going to do anything new? Try to get out of your comfort zone and give it a go!

I'll have a heart attack if I do this
The chances of having a heart attack are extremely remote. If you're at all concerned about any aspect of your health then consult your doctor before embarking on an exercise programme.

I don't have time
If you were told you had a year to live, would you watch television for six hours a night? Would you be thinking non-stop about food?

Evaluate how important you really are, and the base you need to live the life you love. Other aspects of our lives are important but having a strong foundation of self-belief to work from is a very powerful tool, and in Chapter 11 you'll find more on strengthening your inner self. Set your own path and don't follow everyone else; it's time to get inventive. When it's about an issue that you are really committed to, there's no stopping you, so make the time for the important things like getting physical.

It costs too much
You can always start with an exercise video at home, or walking in the neighbourhood. It doesn't cost anything to walk twice to the letterbox or take a flight of stairs. In fact, you could save money if you walked the kids to school or biked to work.

Now we have had a look at some of the reasons for getting active and how to overcome the barriers to exercise, let's move on to see how you can get activity into your daily life and implement a practical programme. In the next two chapters you'll find plenty of ways to take action.

9

TAKING ACTION

It's time to have a look at the level of activity that's right
for you. If you have a pre-existing medical condition or are
concerned about your health, you are advised to consult
your doctor before embarking on any exercise programme,[1] particularly if you:

❖ Have not exercised seriously for over a year.

❖ Are obese.

❖ Have high blood pressure.

❖ Take any prescribed medication.

❖ Are a smoker.

❖ Are over 40 years of age.

Activity is very important in the lifelong maintenance of
your weight. It also keeps us fit, healthy and able to enjoy
life to the full with our friends and family.

If you feel unwell or sustain injury as you start exercising, stop and seek medical advice.

HOW ACTIVE ARE YOU NOW?
You need to determine what level of fitness you're at now,
in order to calculate accurately your starting point.

Little or No Activity
You're at the beginning of the journey and need to see
through the fog of inertia to your destination: a full and

active life. You will see significant benefits in your life very quickly once you get started. You will find that daily activities, such as walking up stairs, carrying the shopping or running for the bus, become easy and manageable. Begin simply by getting activity into your daily life, and progress from here. Read on for ideas and see Chapter 10 for specific programmes.

Starting to Become Active
If you're already making activity a part of your daily routine, then this is wonderful, but it may be time to think about a more structured programme that involves activities such as walking, cycling or swimming. You have planted the seeds of an active lifestyle already and will be able to progress from here, using the practical programmes outlined in the next chapter.

Well on Your Way
You have some regular activity in your life as well as having started a structured exercise programme. Well done: this is a great achievement and you should be proud of yourself. Your aim should be to exercise to a moderate level of activity for at least 30 minutes on at least three to four occasions a week. Once you have managed this, you may wish to begin building up to a more vigorous level of activity on some occasions for 45–60 minutes, and making exercise more frequent.

Right up There
You're exercising on most days of the week for 45–60 minutes and regularly include some vigorous activity in your life. Congratulations – you are at a supreme level of fitness! Keep up the good work. Stay motivated and encourage others to exercise with you, spreading your enthusiasm. Make sure you aim for a comfort level that suits your life and the level of activity you are working to.

GETTING GOING

There are a few basic considerations before you really get going on your new lifestyle plan.

❖ Do less than you think you can initially and don't be too over-ambitious; setting goals that are not achievable will just set you up for failure.

❖ Build up slowly and gradually and start at a level that suits you, even if this is just a short walk or jogging session. Your initial aim, though, should be to build up to the equivalent of walking for at least 30 minutes (or even two 15-minute sessions) on at least five days of the week.

❖ Gradually extend some of your sessions to 45 to 60 minutes and build up to a more vigorous level of activity.

❖ Put more activity into your daily routine: walk up stairs, wash the car by hand, go shopping on foot, walk the dog, do the gardening.

❖ Reduce the amount of time you spend in inactive leisure pursuits such as watching television and replace these sedentary activities with more active pursuits.

❖ Be safe and use your common sense when developing your personal programme. Remember to make activity and exercise as enjoyable as possible by choosing what suits you.

❖ Begin by doing slightly more activity than you usually do, and building steadily. For example if you work on the eighth floor, start by getting the lift to the seventh floor and walking up the last flight of stairs. Then add on one more floor as soon as you feel up to it until you are walking up all the stairs to your office at the beginning of each day. As you build confidence you will be able to increase the amount you do.

❖   There will be days where you will have aching muscles
       or will feel tired. If this is the case have a rest and
       then continue with the exercise the next day. If you
       find you need a break from the more strenuous
       exercise, do some stretches, do a gentle walk or try
       some yoga. Once you feel ready to get back into your
       more active routine then do so, perhaps at a more
       gentle rate, and try to build slower next time or
       change what aspects of the exercise you increase.

To be effective your exercise needs to be steady and
sustained. If you can only do a few minutes on the first
day, that is absolutely great; it's all progress in the right
direction.

WHAT RATE SHOULD I BE WORKING AT?
When you start your programme, build up to a ten-minute
bout at a steady and sustained pace. Then go to 20
minutes, then 30, and ultimately aim for 45–60 minutes.
You will soon find it easy to sustain this level of exercise.
    Ideally you do need a bit of 'huff and puff', but you
should still be able to hold a conversation while you
exercise, otherwise you may well be overdoing things.
Working from the continuum as shown below, aim for a
level of about six or seven.

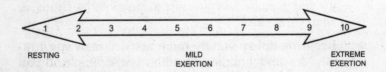

| 1 | 2 | 3 | 4 | 5 | 6 | 7 | 8 | 9 | 10 |

RESTING   MILD   EXTREME
                        EXERTION   EXERTION

WHAT TO WEAR
What you wear will depend on where you're going and
what you're doing. One good general tip is that if your legs
chafe together, apply a protective cream such as Vaseline.
Also you can wear close-fitting stretchy pants to stop the

skin rubbing. If the problem persists, your pharmacist could suggest alternative creams.

At Home
You can wear what you want in the privacy of your own home. The best choice is loose stretch-cotton clothing that you can perspire in.

At the Gym
Again, wear what's comfortable – shorts and T-shirt, a tracksuit or the latest trendy gear. It helps to be organised: keep a set of clothes in a drawer or a bag so you can just grab them.

In the Pool
You'll need a good pair of swimming goggles. If you're intent on pool aerobics, consider investing in a pair of aqua shoes, which can certainly improve the grip. Buying swimwear can be embarrassing if you need a larger size. If there's no specialised stockist nearby, contact a dressmaker to make you something you feel comfortable wearing, investigate the Internet, or purchase via a mail-order catalogue.

Cycling
Always wear a helmet and protective clothing. Wear suitable reflective gear at night, and when it's cold and wet wear a jacket and thermals; on a sunny day use a high-protection suncream. Buy a water bottle that straps onto the bike so you can keep drinking as you cycle and can keep yourself hydrated.

Walking and Running
Wear a good-quality pair of flexible trainers with an arch support and comfortable heel counter. When it's hot and sunny, wear a hat and high-protection suncream, take plenty of water and dress in cool clothing.

EXERCISE OPTIONS

Whether it's as informal as washing the car, or as structured as aqua jogging classes, there are numerous ways to get regular exercise.

Lifestyle

If you don't want to join a class or a gym, get creative in your daily life. Here are some suggestions:

❖ Walk along the beach.

❖ Spring-clean the house.

❖ Do the gardening and enjoy the fresh air.

❖ Dance around the house.

❖ Mow the lawn.

❖ Ask a friend to meet you for a walk.

❖ Get yourself a dog and take it for regular walks.

❖ Offer to walk the neighbour's dog.

❖ Take the stairs instead of the lift.

❖ Park 5 minutes' walk from work or the shops.

❖ Cycle or walk to work.

❖ Make socialising with friends more active (playing golf, tenpin bowling or dancing).

❖ Walk up and down the stairs ten times.

If you have children:

❖ Go for a walk instead of waiting in the car while they're attending sport or a class.

❖ At sports games, walk around the field instead of standing on the sideline.

❖   Join in where possible and maybe even coach a team
      or manage a team and be physically active.

❖   Play active games such as tag, hide and seek or
      soccer.

❖   Go for a walk or run with your child in the pushchair.

One of the times women can be very conscious of their
weight is after having a baby. When you meet with the
antenatal group, suggest a walk around the block or do a
stretching class together. It can be a bit of a giggle.

   If you are retired:

❖   Find a group who want to walk.

❖   Watch the grandchildren play sport and get involved.

❖   While sitting, paddle your feet, stretch your arms
      above your head, turn your neck from side to side,
      brace your knees to get the thigh muscles going.

Home-based Activities
Your body is a natural weight to exercise against and it
doesn't cost you anything. Use what's in your home to
exercise – chairs, stairs, walls, floor space. In Chapter 10
you'll find an exercise plan specifically for keeping fit at
home. You could also borrow some exercise books from
the library, or hire an exercise video.

Joining a Gym
This can be daunting the first time, but don't be put off;
gyms are no longer just for slim aerobics fans! Phone
round the gyms and make a time to visit. Here are some
questions you might ask.

❖   Do they have good showering and changing facilities,
      a sauna and a jacuzzi?

❖ Do they have a good range of aerobics classes to suit all levels?

❖ Do they have fully trained instructors who can customise a programme and show you how to use the equipment?

❖ What is the price? Is there a free trial period?

❖ Is there a quiet time to try out the equipment?

Don't be pushed into buying a membership on the first visit. Take your time and choose the right gym for you.

There is a wide range of equipment to get familiar with. For weightlifting you can use machines, or lift free weights. For cardiovascular training you can walk or run on the treadmill, and control how much you do. The cross-trainer requires a cross-country skiing action; on the stepper you make a high stepping action; and you can strengthen the muscles in your arms, back and legs on the rowing machine. You can do a variety of exercise on a large Swiss ball, which is great for muscle strengthening. Don't worry that it will break under your weight, as there is usually an extra valve to prevent this.

Aerobics Classes
Find out before you go which is the best type of class for you, as different gyms use different names. If you're a beginner, be aware that most in the class will have been attending for some time. Go early and introduce yourself to the instructors. Ask them for advice. Work at your own level and don't feel you have to stay for the whole class.

Is the Pool for You?
Tell the pool attendant if this is your first time, particularly if you're not confident in the water. You don't have to swim lengths of freestyle at a furious pace. Consider some of the following:

❖ Aqua jogging, where you wear a buoyancy belt. If you're concerned it might not fit, ask the assistant if you can go to a private changing room to try it on. Aqua jogging allows you to walk/jog while buoyed by the water, which takes the stress off your joints. It's also great for pregnant women or the elderly.

❖ Pool walking – many pools these days now have a lane for very slow swimmers or walkers. Once you're used to walking you may wish to progress to kicking lengths using a flutter board, playing in the pool, or swimming breaststroke, backstroke or freestyle.

❖ Aqua aerobics classes are a good way to build your water confidence in a safe environment. Again, tell the instructor if it's your first time so he or she can keep an eye on you. Always know that you are in control and you don't have to do every exercise or stay for the whole class.

❖ If you're not yet confident enough to get involved in a class, try doing some resistance work with floats on your own. The instructors at the pool will be able to give you advice on this.

OVERCOMING SETBACKS
Once you're in a regular routine, you'll still need to keep up the positive self-talk: look back over the suggestions in Chapter 8. Take care not to slip back into old habits such as eating as a reward, or thinking negative thoughts.

A LIFELONG SOLUTION
Activity is very important in terms of a lifelong solution to losing weight and keeping the weight off. It is also important to keep us fit and healthy so we are at much reduced risk of disease and are able to enjoy life to the full with our friends and family.

Think about what your starting level is and work forwards from there to a level that suits you best. Choose activities that you find enjoyable and are comfortable with, whether this is just getting more active in terms of your daily routines, working out at home, or visiting a local gym or pool.

Exercise must be fun in order for you to keep at it, so there may be a period of experimentation for a while whilst you find what you really like.

In terms of the actual programmes to follow, Chapter 10 will now go through some of the practical activity programmes, building up your activity from a very basic level to a more advanced level, so read on and get ready to get going.

10

INDIVIDUAL PROGRAMMES

Adjust these programmes to meet your needs. Ensure you listen to your body, resting when tired, and doing more when energised. Start slowly and don't expect too much of yourself: you don't want to burn out in the first week.

Begin by warming and stretching, then embark on the activity itself, extending the time as you get fitter. Do the exercises on alternate days at first, and progress to a daily routine if you can; it doesn't take too much time. Always finish with a cool-down.

Choose a combination of any of the exercises given in this chapter or add more of your own. Choose those that you enjoy, in order to keep at it. You might like to swim twice a week, walk twice a week and have one game of tennis or badminton, for example. Put together a selection that suits you and your lifestyle.

WARM-UP/COOL-DOWN

At the start of any routine you need to warm up the muscles properly to reduce the risk of injury, and afterwards to cool down. Hold each stretch for ten seconds and repeat three times. Move slowly into a stretch and hold without bouncing at the end. Alternate with left and right sides of the body.

Calf Stretch
Place hands on a wall, both feet facing forward, front foot
about 10cm (4 inches) from wall. Extend one leg back, heel
on the floor, and keep straight. Repeat with back leg bent.

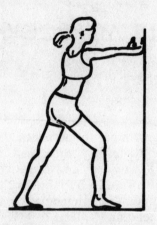

Hamstring Stretch
Place right leg on low-level chair or step. Bend the left
knee and gently stretch forward at the pelvis.

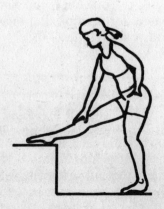

Quad Stretch

Hold onto a wall for balance. Stand on one foot and bend the other foot behind. Bend knee up behind you.

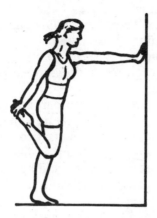

Arm Stretch

Stretch arms across body, holding with the opposite hand.

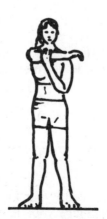

You are now ready to move onto the strengthening and stamina exercises.

STRENGTHENING EXERCISES

Strengthening exercises are designed to strengthen your muscles to give you extra tone. With all the strengthening exercises, remember to move slowly and if you develop any pain then you should reduce or eliminate the exercise and seek professional help. The following exercises can be carried out easily in the comfort of your own home. Alternatively you may wish to go along to a gym – most gyms will put together a programme of strengthening activities for you.

Start on alternate days and progress to doing the routine daily if you can; it doesn't take too much time. As you begin to get stronger, you can start to increase the resistance by using your weight in a different position, as indicated in the exercise, or by adding a handheld weight (these can be purchased from most good sports shops and are relatively inexpensive).

For all the exercises below, start with one set of ten repetitions. As you get stronger work your way up to doing three sets of ten repetitions each time.

Stomach

This exercise will tighten the important muscles on top of your stomach. Lie down and place your hands on the outside of your hips, fingers pointing downwards. Move your thumbs to the inside of your hip bone. Squeeze your stomach muscles in as you pull your tummy-button down towards the floor. You should feel the tummy muscle working under your fingers. Hold the squeeze for five seconds, then release. Repeat ten times and work your way up to three sets of ten repetitions.

Sit-ups

Lie on your back and bend your knees (don't hook your feet under anything). Place your hands on your head or across your chest. Tighten your stomach muscles by sucking in your tummy-button. Lift your shoulders off the floor, hold for five seconds and lie back slowly. Repeat ten times and work your way up to three sets of ten repetitions.

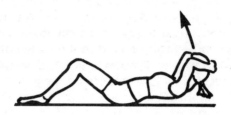

Arm Circles

Stand with your feet hip-width apart and knees slightly bent. Circle your arms backwards ten times, and then forwards ten times. Start with small circling movements and work out to a comfortable circle. As this gets easier you can progress to holding small hand-weights. Work your way up to three sets of ten repetitions in each direction.

Arm circles will mobilise your shoulders. Once you feel ready, you should progress onto strengthening the bicep muscles in your arms. To do this, stand with your feet hip-width apart, knees relaxed and your back in a neutral

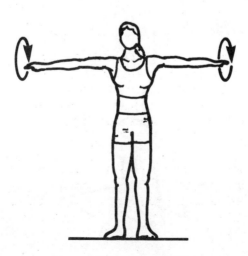

position. Take a small weight in each hand and begin holding your arms straight down next to your body. Slowly bend your elbows, lifting the hands towards the front of the shoulders. Keep the wrists fixed in line with the forearm and the elbow straight below the shoulder. Then, lower your arms slowly until they are straight. Repeat ten times and work your way up to three sets of ten repetitions.

Tip: if you don't have any hand weights around the house then improvise with what's available; for example start with a can of baked beans held in each hand and progress to a 1kg bag of flour in each hand. Eventually, when you are ready, you may wish to invest in a small set of hand weights or join a gym.

Wall Squats
Stand with your back against a wall, your feet shoulder-width apart, and bend to a comfortable squat. Hold for five seconds and return to standing. Repeat ten times and work your way up to three sets of ten repetitions. You could progress to holding small hand-weights, outstretching your arms in front.

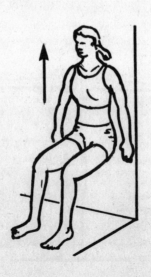

Butt-busters

Lie on your side and bend your lower leg to a 90° angle behind you. Lift the top leg about 30cm (1 ft) off the floor. Hold for five seconds, then lower. Repeat ten times then turn over and do the exercise on the other leg. You may wish to progress to small weights strapped around your ankle. Work your way up to three sets of ten repetitions.

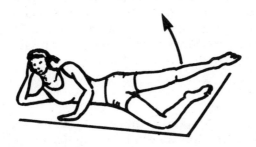

Back Strengthener

Lie on your stomach with your arms stretched out in front of you. Lift your opposite arm and leg off the floor at the same time and hold for ten seconds. Lower your arm and leg slowly to the floor and repeat with the other arm and leg.

Repeat ten times on each side and work your way up to three sets of ten repetitions.

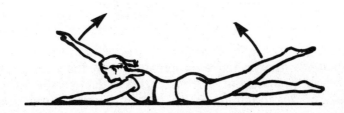

STAMINA EXERCISES

Below are some six-week starter programmes for increasing your stamina by walking, power-stepping, stair-stepping, cycling, swimming or jogging. You may wish to include other activities such as aerobics, badminton, tennis, golf or football. For team games, try to rope in your family or friends.

Start slowly with the stamina exercises but aim to build up to 30 minutes or more at least five times a week. Eventually, you should be able to do 45 minutes or more at a time. A regular exercise programme will help you keep off those excess pounds for the rest of your life.

Walking

Don't be too ambitious at first – if you are a beginner, just walk short distances on gentle terrain. If you find you get tired take your mobile phone and ask a friend to collect you, or call a taxi or take a bus back.

Warm-up/cool-down: 5 minutes walking slowly	
Week	**Minutes of walking**
1	5
2	10
3	15
4	20
5	30–40
6	40–50

Progress to walking further in the same time, walking up a hill or with weights, or power-walk by pumping the arms and really marching with the legs. Gradually extend the time by five to ten minutes a week until you can walk for one to two hours at a moderate pace.

Power-stepping
Power-stepping involves standing on one spot and moving
your arms and legs in a walking/marching action. If at
first you find it too difficult to lift the legs and swing the
arms, just do one or the other. Continue for about 15
minutes at a time (or as long as you can manage) then
progress to 45 minutes or an hour. Put on your favourite
music to give you some rhythm.

Stairs or Step-box
Once you have mastered power-stepping, progress to
stairs or a step-box. Keep the power-stepping at 45
minutes to an hour but add intervals of steps and stairs,
progressing to only steps or stairs. This means stepping
up and down the bottom stair (or continually walking up
and down the stairs), onto a step or a sturdily built box.
Do half the time leading with one leg, and half with the
other leg. Play some music or watch television while you
work out.

Warm-up: 5 minutes power-stepping	
Week	**Minutes of stair-stepping**
1	5
2	10
3	15
4	20
5	25
6	30
Cool-down: 5 minutes slow stepping	

Progress by holding hand-weights or raising the height
of the box.

Cycling

Cycle on an exercise bike, mountain bike or pushbike. You can change the intensity of the workout by altering your speed, the amount of resistance, or the gear level on the bike. Initially do as for walking and go for flat terrain. Bike round a short track several times, or out from home just a short distance.

Warm-up/cool-down: 5 minutes cycling slowly	
Week	**Minutes of cycling**
1	5
2	10
3	15
4	20
5	25
6	30

Progress by five minutes a week until you are cycling for 45 minutes to an hour. Then build intensity by going further in the same time. If on a mountain bike or pushbike, add some hill work.

Pool-based Activity

A workout in the pool can be as gentle or as vigorous as you wish. Start with some gentle aqua jogging or aqua aerobics and progress to swimming.

If you feel nervous do let the pool attendant know. Check how deep the pool is; if you're not confident in deep water then try swimming widths or half-lengths of the pool. Use the swimming stroke you're most comfortable with. If you need the help of a float, take along your own or ask for one at the pool. Try breaststroke or paddling to start with, then work your way up to front crawl, which is a more difficult and energetic stroke. Swim to your own comfort level or ability and use the table below as a rough guide.

Continue to add five more lengths each week, aiming for a session of 45 to 60 minutes. Time yourself each week. To build intensity, aim to swim the total number of lengths in less time.

Warm-up/cool-down: swim 2 lengths slowly	
Week	**Lengths of pool**
1	5
2	10
3	15
4	20
5	25
6	30

Jogging
Jogging is more demanding, so don't try it until you have achieved a reasonable level of fitness. Initially, keep walking for 45 minutes to an hour, but add in intervals of jogging. Eventually you may be jogging continuously.

Warm-up: 5 minutes brisk walking	
Week	**Minutes of jogging**
1	5
2	10
3	10–15
4	15–20
5	20–25
6	25–30
Cool-down: 5 minutes slow walking	

Progress by jogging the whole time, extending the time, or running up more hilly terrain.

INJURY

Prevention is the best policy, so warm up and cool down properly, and wear the appropriate shoes and gear, especially if special equipment is needed. Injuries such as aching shins could be due to overdoing it, or not having the correct footwear. Exercise at your level and ability, particularly if you are playing in a team sport; we all have the potential to become competitive and push ourselves too far. If you are unfortunate enough to suffer an injury, follow these first-aid steps:

❖   Rest and elevate the limb.

❖   Apply ice for ten minutes every two hours for two days.

❖   Compress and support the injury with an elastic bandage.

❖   Exercise by moving gently, but not to the point where it is painful.

Work slowly back into your exercise programme. You may be able to change the activity, for example from walking to swimming. If the pain is considerable, or if swelling and pain persists, see a doctor or physiotherapist.

ILLNESS

The saying that a hard workout 'blows away the cobwebs' does not apply when you are physically unwell. Listen to your body at all times. If you don't feel well, don't exercise.

PUTTING THE PLAN TOGETHER

The information in this chapter can be used to put together a practical programme that suits your own fitness level and lifestyle. It is not prescriptive so use the information as a general guide only, and get into action with the type and level of activity that suits you.

11

YOUR INNER SELF

Achieving inner happiness means you won't need to use food as a crutch. Also, you won't always be avoiding responsibility for your own happiness, with thoughts like, 'If only I could lose a stone I'd feel better.' Not only that, but by overcoming your own barriers to happiness and by losing weight you will be a stronger and healthier person able to enjoy life to the full. Food will become something you eat when you are hungry, something you appreciate and enjoy.

To achieve this level of freedom, you have to work on yourself. Once you are more able to enjoy who you are, you will experience more fulfilling relationships with your family, your friends, work, community and then the world.

First, there has to be a base to work from, and this chapter is all about achieving a sense of balance and inner peace. Most of our lives are spent in our minds – at any time we can choose how we think and even feel. The aim is to gain that sense of control, firstly over yourself, then over your eating habits and your body.

LOVING YOURSELF ...
One of the first steps is to realise that you are a wonderful and valuable person just as you are. Many of us get caught up in day-to-day matters such as chores that need doing, deadlines to meet, and dealing with the kids. Of course, this is important, but we do need to sit back now and again and focus on our 'core self'. This is who we really

are, and the values we want to live our lives by, and it's different for each of us. Have a think about where you're heading in your life. What is important to you now? What do you want to retain or change? It helps to get in touch with this aspect of yourself and the things that matter to you.

Understanding your spiritual side can ultimately help you to manage your weight successfully. Have the belief that you can succeed in what you set out to do, and that you can achieve harmony of mind, body and spirit. Admit when you get it wrong and learn from your mistakes. Don't be too hard on yourself: no one is perfect. Don't chastise yourself about the past – accept it, release it, and move on. Follow your gut instinct when it comes to making important decisions in your life, including how best you can manage your weight.

Life is about choices. Be powerful in your life and make the choices that are right for you now.

... AND OTHERS

It's said that love makes the world go round, and certainly the love in our lives contributes a great deal to our happiness. Have a think about the different forms of love, and identify what is important to you in terms of giving and receiving love:

❖   A smile from a neighbour.

❖   An understanding glance from a friend.

❖   A hug from your kids.

❖   Sharing a great adventure.

❖   Affection from your partner.

❖   An ecstatic greeting from your dog.

Think of ways to increase the love in your life and to enhance your own level of happiness.

STRESS

In this busy world we are all frantically rushing around trying to achieve much more than can be fitted into a normal day. Our stress levels can go through the roof. You may find you turn to food as a way of coping.

One of the main problems with stress is that biologically we are geared up for what's termed the 'fight or flight' response. When our ancestors were faced with danger it was usually in the form of a ferocious wild animal. The choice would have been to fight the animal or to run away, and this is where the term comes from. When faced with stress we produce adrenaline, which prepares our body for action, increasing our pulse and breathing rate.

Of course some level of stress is beneficial, providing us with challenge and excitement, but if we have too much stress we can suffer adverse symptoms including: difficulty sleeping, high blood pressure, anxiety, depression, feelings of panic, dizziness, shortness of breath, poor concentration, no appetite, eating problems.

If the stress is severe and long term, with symptoms such as high blood pressure and depression, you should seek medical advice. Milder levels can be managed with the techniques outlined here. The aim is to cope in other ways than excessive eating.

COPING STRATEGIES

As well as reading through the techniques outlined here, you can also go back to Chapter 3 for other suggestions on looking after yourself.

Exercise

Regular exercise is a wonderful way to relieve stress; it can help you to burn off any extra energy and feel relaxed (see Chapters 8, 9 and 10). You may even find you sleep better. Remember, stress is extremely bad for your health and often can lead to overeating and an exacerbation of weight problems. If you're following the exercise programmes you'll find that exercise is a fantastic coping strategy.

Laughter

Laughter is great medicine and can make you feel really good about yourself. When was the last time you had a real belly-laugh? Have a think about what makes you throw your head back and laugh. Is it seeing a good comedy film? Dancing with abandon? The children being silly, or even being silly yourself? Don't be too reserved, or worry about what people might think of you. Make time for the things in life that make you laugh.

Time with Others

If you're a loner then you may need time with others to help release tension and gain a broader perspective on life. This is particularly likely if you're single and live alone. Think about inviting friends over for a meal or taking up some new hobbies that involve meeting others. Sporting interests are particularly good as you not only improve your social contact but you burn up that extra energy and help to alleviate stress.

Solitary Time

Do you continually have to have people around you? If you do then you are not taking the time to get in tune with yourself. Consider having some 'time out', even if it's just for half an hour or a day. If you live in the countryside you might like to find yourself a nice quiet spot to retreat to locally if you can, maybe a quiet wooded area or a local beach. If you live in a busy city you might like to find a place within your own house or apartment that you can retire to in order to be on your own; it might be the bathroom for a long soak in the bath, or it might be the garden. Quieten your mind and focus on relaxation. The techniques discussed later in this chapter will help you get started on this path.

Get Food Back on Track

If you have turned to food, aim to get back on track as soon as possible and don't be too harsh on yourself. We are all human and can make mistakes. Don't stress about the fact that you have just demolished a large bag of potato chips or a whole packet of biscuits. Just learn from your mistakes and think about what prompted you to eat these foods and how you can avoid such prompts in the future. Look at getting your food intake back on track. Have a look at Chapter 3 for more information in this area.

Pamper Yourself
Find activities to get involved in that make you feel special. There is lots of information on this in Chapter 3 so have a look for the ideas that suit you and fit into your life.

RELAXATION
We've all suffered from an overactive mind, busily thinking of a thousand things at once when we're extremely stressed. Quietening your mind can be a challenge initially, but there are some very useful techniques to help you relax, achieve focus and control, and avoid the temptation of reaching for the biscuit tin.

Aim to relax each day if you can, even if it's just for ten minutes. If you can spare as long as an hour for relaxation though, that's even better. There are four key techniques that you can use to help yourself relax: tension and relaxation; colour and light; imagination and visualisation; and mind focus. These techniques are described below.

Setting the Scene
Initially it is important to set the scene to relax. Create a quiet peaceful environment. Try out some of the following:

❖   Take the phone off the hook.

❖   Tidy the room.

❖   Light a candle.

❖   Light some incense sticks or a fragranced oil burner.

❖   Have a hot bath or shower.

❖   Wear comfortable clothes – nothing tight.

❖   Play quiet peaceful music.

❖   Try out the different chairs or the floor and see where you are comfortable.

❖   Decide whether you prefer sitting or lying.

Breathing
Once you are settled, slowly breathe in through your nose and out through your mouth for about three or four breaths. Use your diaphragm, at the base of your ribs. Relax your upper chest and feel the diaphragm muscle move out as you breathe in, and in as you breathe out. Then breathe at your own rate and rhythm throughout the relaxation.

Tension and Relaxation
Focus on each of the main muscle groups, working your way through the body. Tighten and feel the tension in the muscle, holding for five seconds. Release completely, allowing the tension to drain away. Do this right through your body, working upwards in the following order: toes, feet, calves, thighs, buttocks, stomach (pull in), shoulders (pull back), arms, fists (clench), jaw (clench), eyes (screw up), face (scrunch up).

Colour and Light
Imagine a candle is glowing just below your chest, on your diaphragm. Concentrate on the light, how warm and soft it is. Let the light filter up round your heart, head and shoulders, then drift down your arms and legs. Take the light around your body in a protective and loving way. Become aware of your body. Is there any area of tension? Can you feel or see a colour connected to the area of

tension? Surround the area with a warm glowing light and feel the tension ease.

Imagination and Visualisation
You can go anywhere, any time with your imagination, so use it in a positive way. You could imagine one of the following scenarios, or create your own. Memorise the sequences below, or read them onto a tape and play them to yourself (see below).

The Tropical Island
You're walking along a beautiful golden beach, with a perfect blue sky and the hot sun shining down on you. The waves roll gently onto the shore as sparkles of light shimmer on the water. You feel the warmth of the sun on your cheek and smell the fresh salty sea air. There is no one else in sight.

As you amble down the beach, you come across a small rowing boat with two wooden oars. You pick up the oars and push the boat into the water, and then hop in. Gently and leisurely you begin to row out to sea, taking in the scenery as you go, feeling the cool breeze on your face. A group of dolphins starts to follow your boat, frolicking in the water. You lie back in the boat and watch the dolphins at play; you are in no rush. As the boat drifts out to sea you spot a tropical island in the distance, and you pick up the oars and begin to row towards it. Once there you pull the boat onto the shore and lie down on the white sand. Feel the warmth of the sun, enjoy the tranquil atmosphere, listen to the waves splashing onto the shore, and drift into a state of deep relaxation. Stay there for as long as you please. When you're ready, wander down to the boat and row back.

The Forest Walk

You're walking along a narrow, winding path surrounded by beautiful dense forest. Look at the different-shaped trees and bushes as you saunter along. See the dew on the leaves sparkle; listen to the birds singing as you pass by. Watch as an array of brightly coloured butterflies flutters in front of you; see the beautifully vivid colours of their wings against the deep green of the surrounding forest. As the path begins to wander upwards you move higher and you begin to feel weightless, almost as though you are floating. There is a wooden bench in front of you. Stop and sit down, and look at the stunning view in front of you: forest, sand, deep blue sea; vivid green, stark white and deep blue. Feel the gentle wind blowing through your hair as you take a deep breath and breathe out all the tension from your body. Relax here for as long as you wish before strolling back down the path.

The Old House
You see an old wooden fence and beyond it a big old brick house. You walk up the rose-lined path to the front door, which is slightly open. As you push the door it creaks loudly. You step into a large hallway, at the end of which is a big winding staircase. Your footsteps echo on the floor as you walk towards the stairs and begin your ascent. As you reach the top of the staircase you see a number of doors in front of you. You open the nearest door, which opens into a library. The shelves are laden with old books of every size and colour imaginable. You gaze around the room, drinking in the culture and history. You begin to feel tired and decide to find a bed to lie down on. As you leave the library you're drawn to a large oak door with a brass handle. You walk forwards slowly and open the door. Inside the room is a large four-poster bed with lace-embroidered sheets. Your body feels heavy; you walk towards the bed and lie down. You close your eyes and feel at peace with yourself. Stay in this place for as long as you like. Keep your mind empty and focus on achieving a deep sense of relaxation. When you feel ready, open your eyes and rise from the bed. Leave the bedroom, walk down the stairs and leave the house, closing the door behind you. Walk towards the gate, knowing that you can return at any time to this house.

Mind Focus
If you find it difficult to focus your mind, one useful technique is to count to ten slowly. Think of the number ten as being a complete state of relaxation. Now begin counting from number one. See the number one in your mind's eye; focus totally on that number as you take a deep breath in and a deep breath out. Feel the tension flow out

of your body slowly and gently. Now see the number two: you are a little more relaxed already. Breathe in and out slowly again, slipping further into a state of relaxation. Feel your mind quieten and your body relax. Keep counting in this way until you reach number ten. If your mind begins to drift, start counting again from number one.

Some people like to use a candle to focus the mind. Sit comfortably with a candle in front of you. Concentrate on the candle and as you watch the flame flicker, clear your mind completely of any thoughts. Just give the candle all your attention as you feel yourself unwind and relax. If your mind drifts, pull back to the light of the candle.

Your own Relaxation Tape
You may like to make a relaxation tape yourself, using the techniques described above. Think about the method that works best for you, and how long you want to spend relaxing. Buy a blank tape of the correct length, and then write yourself a script. You might like to tape-record the sea or the noises you hear in a wood, so you have some nature sounds in the background to focus on during the pauses. Time yourself and make sure you talk slowly and have sufficient pauses. You may need to try out a few versions before you get one that's right for you.

Now that you know what a quiet mind feels like, with practice you will be able to get into this peaceful state quite easily. Use the techniques whenever you need to during the day, as a way of alleviating stress and taking your mind off food, or at night to help you sleep. Don't forget to put time aside for yourself on a regular basis, for your own physical and mental well-being.

12

MUTUAL MOTIVATION

We live in a society obsessed with being thin. In fact, obesity has been described as the last remaining socially acceptable form of prejudice.[1] Fear of fat is deeply engrained in our culture; it has even been reported in the USA that many kids believe being fat is the same as being cursed.[2] So where does this attitude come from? Well, the media and the fashion and beauty industry are partly to blame. *Playboy* centrefolds and Miss America contestants have become thinner in recent years[3] and many adverts portray stick-thin women who lack feminine curves and are significantly below their ideal weight. More recently, we have seen a backlash against this trend with beautiful models of a more realistic weight spread across many fashion pages. Unfortunately though, this is the exception rather than the rule, and we have a long way to go in changing the attitudes of this 'fat-phobic' society.

Although it would be nice to think that attitudes will change, we have to accept this will be a slow process. For now, we need to think about beginning a trend of mutual motivation. This means learning to deal with the anguish and social isolation felt by many of us with weight problems, and with the unenlightened attitudes of others.

You might not be overweight yourself, but want to support your friend or partner as he or she loses weight. The information in this chapter will be useful to share with those going through this weight loss programme, and with others who are giving support.

HANDLING CRITICISM

People are often involved in their own problems and sometimes make insensitive and thoughtless comments. It can be difficult not to believe the judgments other people make about you. However, once you get over the initial shock of how cruel some people can be, remind yourself that they can only be as nice to you as they are to themselves: they must be having a pretty miserable life if they can be so nasty.

If you can evaluate what sort of person you're dealing with, you have a better idea of how to address their attitudes. Here are some common traits among those who make negative comments.

Insulting

Some people make comments so thoughtless it takes your breath away. Here are some genuine examples.

❖ 'You're going to die young if you don't lose weight.'

❖ 'Just stop eating – it's that simple. Don't open your mouth.'

❖ 'Maybe your brother and sister will love you if you lose weight.'

❖ 'Just think what it will be like to be normal.'

❖ 'When is your baby due?'

❖ 'You don't need to eat that, do you?'

❖ Airline steward, loudly: 'I'll just go and get you a seatbelt expander, dear.'

❖ Dancer: 'The reason I never ask you to dance is that I find it awkward to dance with big women.'

❖ Shop assistant: 'We don't stock anything that big.'

There are two ways to deal with these types of people:

❖   Confront them, *or*

❖   Make yourself safe by moving away or trying to ignore their remarks.

How you respond will also depend on how close you are to them. With a friend, you may wish to front up to him or her and explain how you feel. With a stranger in a bar, just ignore it. The most important thing to remember is that you mustn't be intimidated into negative action: if an insulting comment means you don't go dancing, then you have given in.

Inquisitive
Some people will question you intensely about what you're doing, in order to find fault with it, or to offer their own advice. They always know best: you will probably not be following the right diet or exercise plan! The world is full of such people, who are often uninformed, so ask what their opinions are based on and challenge them if appropriate. You can turn an inquisitive person into an ally; they often have your best interests at heart, so include them in your strategy on losing weight and explain why you're doing it. Start with positive comments, thanking them for their interest in your wellbeing, and then explain the issues from your own perspective. You may have to accept, however, that you can't change other people's opinions – but don't be swayed from your own path.

Passive
These types appear not to care less what you do. Examine the reasons why you may want them to take an interest. With your partner or a friend, explain why you would like their support and what they can do to help you. It may just be that they are not aware that you have a problem or are in need of support. If they continue to be disinterested, however, find someone else to support you.

Self-absorbed
Somehow, these people manage to turn your weight
problem into being about them. A friend may say, 'I
can't go to the pool if you won't go', or a partner may
say, 'Get things into perspective, after all, I deal with a
ten million pound budget and you're worried about a
silly craving for chips.'

Try to be supportive of others, but explain that it has
to be reciprocated. It should be a mutually positive
situation.

SEEKING SUPPORT

Think about the kind of support that works for you and
what you need from those who love you and care about
you. Learn to communicate the way in which you want to
be treated. Maybe hearing that you look slimmer really
inspires you to continue, or maybe you don't want attention drawn to your weight. Be realistic in what you ask of
others and be careful about how you handle difficult
situations with your friends or your partner. With the
rhythm of life, friendships come and go. Move on if a
support person is insensitive, rude or unsupportive.

HELPING OTHERS

Some overweight people are quite happy with their weight
as it is. We have to accept and respect this, and love them
as they are. However, for those who do wish to lose weight,
it can be very difficult to get the right balance – what to
say, how to act, when to be caring and when to be firm.
Being there when they explode, or won't talk, or cry for
hours, can be a really difficult process for all involved.
You'll be appreciated for taking the time and energy to
care, and you'll also feel rewarded as you see others
achieve their goals.

Take a look at your own life. Are you happy? Are you
on fire with your life and living passionately? If not, then
re-evaluate your values and lifestyle and work through
your own issues, as the more energy and power you have,

the more support you will be able to give to others. The following points may be useful in helping you to understand and support your friend or partner in his or her efforts to lose weight.

❖ Most of us have a weakness, whether it's smoking or alcohol, spending too much on clothes or an addiction to talk shows. With big people who overeat, their weakness is apparent to everyone and they are judged for it. To help you understand the desire others have to overeat and to enable you to offer support, have a think about what your own weakness is.

❖ Examine your own eating habits and see if they are trying to nurture your food needs. Many women still apply the old adage, 'The only way to a man's heart is through his stomach.' Consider whether one of the ways you give love is by providing unhealthy or excessive food.

❖ If someone you live with is trying to lose weight and has a real weakness for a particular food – cheese, crisps, cakes, ice cream, chocolates – support that person by not buying these foods. You can always eat them when you're out, but having them at home may be too much temptation for the person trying to lose weight.

❖ Always ask about takeaway foods and eating out. It may not be wise to bring a surprise meal of fish and chips home as a treat. A basic principle of weight loss is having a healthy, balanced diet that the whole family can enjoy.

❖ When complimenting someone who is overweight, why not tell them how vivacious, bright and happy they are, how great their nails or hair look, or what a fantastic new outfit they're wearing, rather than drawing attention to their weight.

❖ Don't chastise people you have cooked for if they don't eat everything on their plate. In fact, it might be a good idea to let people serve themselves.

❖ When you invite people to dinner, ask if there are any foods they don't like or if they have any special requirements. Then you're providing an open forum and not treating overweight people differently. Try to provide the type of food they require and don't make their meal different from others'. If you want a dessert, make it a healthy option and let them decide whether to eat some.

❖ People who are trying to lose weight often get fed up with questions such as 'How much weight have you lost?' This is none of your business and just draws attention to the issue.

❖ As a support person your aim is to inspire and motivate, not judge and criticise. This is what is most valued and appreciated. Let the other person talk about weight. Always reinforce the fact that you will provide love, support and friendship unconditionally, which means it doesn't matter what their weight is or how much weight they have or have not lost.

❖ Food addicts can be great manipulators to get their own way. This may involve acting in a childlike manner around food, being coy or flirtatious. Avoid being harsh or bossy but do try to discourage game-playing.

You may be unsure of how to give support. Ask yourself: Is now the right time? How am I going to give support? Am I the right person to do it? We've all made well-intentioned comments that have not been well received. Being overweight is a sensitive issue and a blunt opinion is not always what is sought. The following types of comments are not helpful: 'I've lost so much weight … the way I did it is the only way', 'I think you should go on a diet',

'Have you thought of investing in an exercise machine to lose that extra weight?' 'Hey, that woman over there looks great', 'I would love you more if you were thinner.'

If you're fed up with hearing about food issues from your friend or partner, communicate how you feel in a loving way. Maybe make a pact to say nothing about emotions, food or exercise for a given time. Expand on how you express your love, affection or friendship: trips away, flowers, a gentle hand on the shoulder, coming home early, looking after the kids, a walk along the beach. Make special occasions such as birthdays and anniversaries about affection rather than food.

LOBBYING FOR CHANGE

There are many ways in which we can encourage a better informed and healthier society, and if enough of us do this we may actually start to see some action.

To help change attitudes to the overweight, write to your favourite magazines with suggestions such as: using models to reflect the average woman, who after all is the main reader of the magazine; promoting clothes that are available in larger sizes; including ideas for sewing your own clothes. Ask your local restaurants to include healthy options on the menus and have seating appropriate for larger people. Contact the local school to suggest starting up a 'walking bus', collecting children to walk to school in a group. Ask them to include healthy options on the school lunch menu and in the tuck shop. You could start an action group to set up policies on nutrition and physical activity.

To promote policy changes, write to your Member of Parliament and/or local council suggesting:

❖   More funding for the treatment of weight loss by qualified health professionals.

❖   Environmental policies that promote physical activity, such as safe and well-lit walkways and cycle paths.

❖   Better education in schools on nutrition and basic cooking skills and more physical activity for our school children.

❖   New legislation to crack down more severely on those who make false and misleading claims on weight-loss products.

If enough people start working together, we may slowly begin to change the attitudes of society and generate an environment that is more compassionate and supportive towards those with a weight problem.

13

PUTTING IT ALL TOGETHER

You've now read all the information, advice and ideas on how to lose weight and implement a new way of eating, exercising, and giving and receiving support – not just for a few weeks or a few months, but for the rest of your life. This is a new knowledge base, like a set of tools, ready for you to use. Here is a summary of the key points you need to remember to help keep you on track. Use this as a reminder to yourself at different times, as you progress. You can just dip into this section of the book every six months or so to recap on your new direction in life.

WHY WAIT FOR CHANGE?
Making changes to our lifestyle or eating habits is not easy and that's why we often put things off with silly little excuses like 'I don't have time' or 'It's too hard'. Human beings inherently tend to resist change; it's a well-known phenomenon! We feel comfortable with what we know, with the situations we have surrounded ourselves with.

Lack of time can also be a real problem. Modern society is just full of stressed-out people rushing around trying to cram as much into life as possible: careers, social life, family, friends, community work, other obligations; the list goes on. It is often difficult to imagine where you could possibly find the time to embark on a new lifestyle programme, but the first step is to sit down and really plan out your time well. Is there anything that you are doing that you don't enjoy? Can you give up that particular activity or get some help? Can you streamline your time better by getting more organised?

Think upon this as an exciting new lifestyle and embrace the new choices and changes that you are planning to make in your life with enthusiasm and a quiet knowing that you are on the right track. Make it an adventure that you have never followed to the full before because although change can be daunting and challenging, it can also be exciting and refreshing.

It is now time to take action: you have read this book, you have all the necessary information at your fingertips to make the changes you need to make, and you are now ready to implement a strategy to change your lifestyle and to lose the weight for ever.

Think carefully about the best way forward and start to put in place small gradual changes. Remember you are a strong and powerful person, you can achieve the goals you wish to achieve; it is just a matter of being focused and having the right tools (the information in the power of positive eating strategy) to put the changes into practice.

You can now look forward to making steady achievable changes that will actually work in the long term, rather than following one fad diet after another and seeing your weight yo-yo up and down.

Put Yourself First
We often put the needs of others before our own; women in particular, as nurturers, are often guilty of this. It's good to be unselfish and to help others, but if you're stressed, upset or depressed and seek comfort in food, then you're not in the best position to give to others. So, there is the justification for taking some 'you' time. In the end those around you will also benefit from being with a person who is happier, less stressed and healthier. They can also enjoy a better diet and a more active lifestyle themselves.

No matter what your situation, as a person you are free; free to make the right choices in your life for you. If something in your life is getting in the way of true happiness and causing you to eat for comfort, think about what you can do to change it. It may be a relationship, a job or a set of friends. More information is given on this in Chapter 3, so have a look and remind yourself of the best strategies for coping.

ACHIEVING YOUR GOALS

Your goals must be achievable and sustainable. A target that is too ambitious will only leave you disappointed and losing motivation.

Set yourself little tasks for each day. Each small change will have a positive impact in the right direction. If, for example, you currently eat only one portion of fruit or vegetables each day, to jump up to the recommended five portions a day is a giant leap. Add just one portion a day and work from there. The same applies to exercise. If you're completely inactive, don't expect to go for a long run or aerobics class, or even a long walk. Use the exercise information in Chapter 10 to begin slowly. Just getting up five minutes earlier in the morning to practise some stretching, relaxation exercises or even walking will mean you're moving in the right direction.

Aim to lose weight at a healthy rate and in a way that reduces fat tissue. Look at Chapter 5, where we recommend a weight loss of around 0.25 to 1kg (0.5–2 lb) per week. You may lose weight slightly more quickly at first, then level off a little, but do avoid rapid weight loss. Congratulate yourself on your successes. Tell others, have a party or give yourself a treat!

EMPOWERING YOURSELF

Think of this as the start of a new adventure, a life where you are more in control – of your weight, your health, your activities and your feelings. Believe in yourself and explain to those around you how they can best support you.

Identify your weaknesses and think about strategies to deal with them. Do you have a passion for a particular food such as cheese, chocolate or potato chips? Then don't buy them, and ask your family to avoid bringing them home. Good social support can be one of the factors in successful results for many of us. Have a look again at the information in Chapter 12, and pass it on. At the same time, do be careful of those who are overly opinionated or meddlesome.

POSITIVE EATING

The information in Chapters 5, 6 and 7 will really get you started on the right path to a healthy eating style for you and your family. The food and exercise patterns that are recommended are suitable for your whole family (except for very young children or those with special dietary needs). This will make life easier for you as you don't have to prepare separate meals for yourself, and everyone will benefit from all the health advantages of a good diet and will manage to maintain their weight at a healthy level.

Just remember to get the portion sizes right, have roughly the right amounts of foods through the day and aim for a balance of the different food groups as shown in the balanced plate model described in Chapter 5. Fill up on fruits and vegetables if you feel hungry, and remember those cakes, biscuits and potato chips that are marketed as being '95% fat-free' are not foods that should be eaten in abundance, as they are often high in calories and sugar.

Don't be too hard on yourself and do allow the odd treat; this will make your new eating habits much more sustainable and achievable. Perhaps have a healthy pudding or treat once a week; some delicious recipe ideas for puddings and treats are given in Chapter 7.

The basic key to a healthy diet is just to get the balance right, fill up on those fruits and vegetables and aim to have most of your calories from carbohydrate foods such as bread, rice and pasta, especially wholegrain varieties. Have moderate amounts of lean meat and low-fat dairy products and really focus on keeping your fat intake to a minimum – this is the most concentrated source of calories

– and limiting your intake of high-sugar foods.

Just remember to have the right attitude to your food too: don't become overly obsessed with the calorie content of every morsel that passes through your lips and don't worry about weighing and measuring everything you eat. By just following the basic guidelines outlined in this book you will achieve success.

STAYING ACTIVE

Perhaps one of the most important factors in achieving weight loss is getting active. Scientific studies have found close associations between inactivity and weight gain. For example those who watch lots of television are more likely to be overweight. Of course watching television is not a very sociable pastime either; it is much more fun to go out to the local park and go for a run, or play a game of football, rounders or cricket with the family. If you have the time, a dog can be a great way of getting active, taking it out for long walks each day. Think about what kind of activity suits you, your lifestyle, your friends and your family and implement that activity.

Perhaps the most important thing to remember in terms of activity is that it should be fun. If you absolutely hate jogging or swimming then don't do it. Find something else you enjoy. Remind yourself of all the options that are open to you by looking again at the information in Chapters 8, 9 and 10. Also, don't forget to build up slowly and gradually by setting small and realistic goals.

IF YOU LOSE YOUR WAY

If you feel angry with yourself for doing something wrong you will see yourself as a victim. Stop! Do not chastise yourself, feel sorry for yourself and feel miserable. Do not give up! Take back the power and regain control. You'll achieve nothing by fretting over past mistakes; the past is in the past and you can't change it. It's important, therefore, just to move on with life. You need to feel good about yourself and to build on your self-esteem. How you do this is a very personal issue but it may be that you seek the company of people around you for support, or that you get involved with new activities and develop new interests. If you do make a mistake or have a weak moment, use it as a learning process and think about putting in place safeguards to prevent future relapses.

Think of yourself as a special and unique person who can achieve anything in life simply by focusing on it and devising a plan of action, a series of stepping stones that will get you to your goals. Do not chastise yourself for your failure, rather look upon your successes and think about how you can build on these to achieve what you wish to achieve. It is often said that growth comes from pain and struggle in life. Learn from your past experiences, recognise that you are human and that we all make mistakes and learn lessons then move on. Learn to grow and develop through joy and happiness.

It is important to focus on all your good points and avoid comparing yourself to others. It might be nice to think you could pick out all the perfect bits of different people and acquire those characteristics or traits, but the truth is that's just a fairytale. We are all human and we all have our frailties and faults. We need to learn to live with ourselves and love ourselves for who we are.

Although it is important to learn from those around you, do be careful of those who are overly opinionated without being in possession of the true facts. Use the information in this book as a basis for your lifestyle changes. And don't forget, when people do start to offer their opinion, look at what their qualifications are and how credible a source of information they are. Make sure the changes that you put in place are ones that suit you and fit in with your own lifestyle. It is you, after all, who needs to follow this new dietary and lifestyle regimen.

TRUST YOURSELF
Losing weight and maintaining that weight loss is not easy. That's why there is an endless round of books, videos and

weird and wonderful remedies constantly adorning the shelves of our local shops and booming out of our televisions and radios, promising instant success with no effort. Quick-fix results are a myth we want to believe in and that is why proponents of such remedies make money, preying on our vulnerabilities and insecurities.

You can achieve success, though, by understanding the issues involved and implementing the right strategies for you. Now you have read this book you will have picked up all the key tips and hints for a successful new life. Just remember these things:

❖   You will now be able to implement a new way of eating and living that will benefit you and your family both now and into the future.

❖   You will now have a good level of knowledge on the different fad diets and miracle cures and understand what does and doesn't work, and why.

❖   You will be ready to put in place an action plan to get active, which will be fun and will help burn off those extra calories, resulting in weight loss.

❖   You will have achieved an insight into the psychological factors involved and the factors that motivate change.

❖   You will be able to start putting together a support network through friends and family, and through developing new interests.

14

THE WEBSITE

We really want you to succeed in losing your weight and maintaining that weight loss. You may find that just reading this book is enough to get you started and keep you motivated as you embark on your new lifestyle. However, many of us find an ongoing support network extremely helpful, so we'll be giving you ongoing support and help, if you need it, through our website www. thepowerofpositiveeating.com.

The whole philosophy of the power of positive eating is that this is a brand new approach to weight loss with a new healthy eating and healthy living programme and ongoing support. Most books promoting dietary regimens just sell the book to you and then forget about you. You'll find that you follow these diets for a short time while you are motivated, and then you slip back into the old habits. Support can be one factor that helps sustain long-term weight loss and weight maintenance and that's the idea behind the book and the website package.

You'll be able to log on for all the latest information, advice and support as it becomes available. There will be the chance for you to share your experiences with others; you'll be able to give and receive helpful tips and hints for success.

What have you got to lose? Live a little and take the plunge; we are there for you and you will see that you are not alone. When you hear that others are just like you and your secrets aren't secrets any more, but experiences to learn from, then there is real hope. It is amazing the differences this will make in your life.

ACCESS
If you don't have a computer you can use one at a cyber café, local library, or maybe use a friend's.

NEWSLETTER
A regular online newsletter will keep you informed of the latest news in the world of diet, nutrition and exercise.

TIPS
Find out about the latest food and exercise tips, including new and interesting recipe ideas and different options for getting active.

If you have any exciting ideas that you would like to share with us, please contact us via the website. We will include as many of your good ideas as we can on the website so that others can benefit from your knowledge.

SUCCESS STORIES
Have a look at some of our success stories to inspire and motivate you. You may even like to send a recent picture and a success story of your own. We will do our best to include as many of your success stories as we can.

SUPPORT
You can seek different levels of support, depending on your needs and the amount of time you have to invest. At one end of the spectrum you may just like to dip into the site for information or just have online conversations now and again; alternatively you may wish to get actively involved in setting up and facilitating a support group in your area.

YOUR PROFILE
This is the opportunity for you to tell others about yourself with a collection of online information that will form

a personal profile. Your personal information profile can include basic information such as age, gender, marital status, geographical location and interests. All this is through the anonymity of the Internet. You can even create a nickname if you don't want to give your real name, and the beauty of this system is that your email address is kept confidential and is not known by any of the people online. As you get to know people you may become more confident and can reveal information about yourself if you choose, but you have the opportunity to reveal as much or as little as you like.

You can say what you are hoping to gain from your web experiences, whether simply chatting online, or actually meeting new people in a similar situation to your own. You can set up your own local support networks to keep each other motivated, share your woes and misfortunes, and of course your advice and successes.

ONE-ON-ONE

Getting online is a great way of hooking up with similar people to share experiences about weight problems. You'll unravel the patterns, and learn about food, exercise and your inner self. You may want to take things further by swapping telephone numbers and giving each other support via the telephone.

Ultimately you may wish to meet people face to face. If you do, exercise caution. Don't give out too many personal details before meeting (for example, your address or place of work) and always meet in a public place. Never meet anyone until you have exchanged *landline* telephone numbers (not just mobile numbers) and have spoken at least a couple of times by phone. Tell a friend where you are going, or take a friend with you and make sure other people know who you are meeting and when you will be back for safety reasons. There are some great opportunities out there, but keep yourself secure until you get to know someone.

SUPPORT GROUPS

One of the great features of the power of positive eating approach is the ongoing support and help you will receive from our website at www.thepowerofpositiveeating.com. When trying to lose weight, those who have ongoing support can have a greater chance of success. You can easily set up your own group support network in your area if this is something that would help you. And the great thing is you won't have to pay out money and go through the embarrassment of being weighed each week; you can just meet for a drink in a local café, or can even rendez-vous in a local park.

The first things to decide are:

❖   Do you want to be involved in a support group?

❖   Do you want to set up and facilitate a group, or just go along as a group member?

If you simply want to join a group, then have a look on the website to see if there is anything going on in your area. If not, there may be other local community groups already set up where you live that you could go along to – check out your local library for information.

If you want to set up your own group, think about how you will get the group started.

❖   Put a note on our website at www.thepowerof positiveeating.com.

❖   Put notices at the local bookstore, library or gym.

❖   Invite friends, acquaintances and work colleagues.

Then you will need to think about how you will run the group. You'll need to decide on a venue – this may be in a local coffee shop or health club, or perhaps in someone's house. Decide on the frequency of the group meetings and ensure you start and end on time. Hold a group session when you say you will and be careful not to let people down.

As a facilitator you may be challenged to be inclusive, tolerant and non-critical. You may find people asking you questions and expecting you to have answers. Instead of providing answers and solutions, encourage group members to resolve their own problems by swapping information on food and exercise. Rather than giving advice, and being too dictatorial, you can empower others by asking them 'What do you think the answer is to your situation?' then ask for comments and advice from others in the group. Remember that we all learn from one another.

Suggestions for the group:

* ❖ Sharing their experiences.

* ❖ Reading sections out of the book.

* ❖ Swapping recipes and meal ideas.

* ❖ Exercise during that time, perhaps organise to meet to walk, swim or run.

At the end, thank the members for coming to the group and work together to spread the word about the group and encourage others to join in.

FREQUENTLY ASKED QUESTIONS
You can access helpful information, including answers to frequently asked questions, and email us with questions.

FEEDBACK
Do email us with your reactions to the book and the website. We look forward to your participation.

NOTES

Chapter 1

1. Stunkard, A.J., & J. Sobal, 'Psychological Consequences'. In K.D. Brownell and C.G. Fairburn, *Eating Disorders and Obesity: A Comprehensive Handbook*. The Guilford Press, New York, 1995.

Chapter 2

1. www.iotf.org.
2. Crawford, D., R.W. Jeffery, & S.A. French, 'Can Anyone Successfully Control their Weight? Findings of a Three-year Community-based Study of Men and Women.' *International Journal of Obesity*, 24, 2000: 1107–11.
3. Czajka-Narins, D.M., & E.S. Parham, 'Fear of Fat: Attitudes Toward Obesity'. *Nutrition Today*, January/February 1990: 26–32.
4. Orbach, S., *Fat is a Feminist Issue*. Arrow, London, 1989.
5. Morgan, J.F., 'From Charles Atlas to Adonis Complex – Fat is More Than a Feminist Issue'. The Lancet, 356, 2000: 1372–3.
6. www.iotf.org.
7. Prentice, A., 'Overview of Obesity Management'. *Proceedings of the New Zealand Dietetic Association Conference*, 3, 1998: 42–6.
8. Scottish Intercollegiate Guidelines Network (SIGN), *Obesity in Scotland. Integrating Prevention with*

Weight Management. A National Clinical Guideline Recommended for Use in Scotland. SIGN, Edinburgh, 1996.

Chapter 3

1. British Nutrition Foundation, *Obesity: The Report of the British Nutrition Foundation Task Force.* Blackwell Science, Oxford, 1999.
2. Orbach, S., *Fat is a Feminist Issue.* Arrow, London, 1989.
3. Ni Mhurchu, C., B.M. Margetts, & V.M. Speller, 'Applying the Stages-of-change Model to Dietary Change'. *Nutrition Reviews*, 55, 1, 1997: 10–16.

Chapter 4

1. American Dietetic Association, 'Food and Nutrition Misinformation. Position of the American Dietetic Association'. *Journal of the American Dietetic Association*, 95, 1995: 705–7.
2. Kurtzweil, P., 'How to Spot a Health Fraud'. *FDA Consumer*, November/December 1999: 22–26.
3. Freedman, M.R., J. King & E. Kennedy, 'Popular Diets: A Scientific Review'. *Obesity Research*, 9(1), 2001: 1s–40s.
4. St Jeor, S.T., et al., 'Dietary Protein and Weight Reduction. A Statement for Healthcare Professionals from the Nutrition Committee of the Council on Nutrition, Physical Activity, and Metabolism of the American Heart Association'. *Circulation* 104 (15), 2001: 1869.
5. Foster G.D., Wyatt H.R., Hill J.O., et al. (2003), 'A Randomised Trial of a Low-carbohydrate Diet for Obesity.' *New England Journal of Medicine* 348: 2082–90.
6. Samaha F.F., Iqbal N., Seshadri P., et al. (2003), A Low-carbohydrate as Compared with a Low-fat Diet in Severe Obesity.' *New England Journal of Medicine* 348: 2074–81.

7.   National Institute of Health, National Heart, Lung and Blood Institute, North American Association for the Study of Obesity, *Obesity: The Practical Guide to Identification, Evaluation and Treatment of Overweight and Obesity in Adults*. NIH Publication No. 00–4084, 2000.

8.   D'Adamo, P.J., with C. Whitney, *Eat Right for Your Type*. Putnam, New York, 1996.

Chapter 5

1.   Astrup, A., 'Dietary Strategies for Weight Management – the Importance of Carbohydrates'. *Australian Journal of Nutrition and Dietetics*, 58 (1), 2001: s9–s12.

2.   Food Standards Agency and Institute of Food Research, *McCance and Widdowson's The Composition of Foods*. Sixth summary edition. Cambridge: Royal Society of Chemistry, 2002.

3.   Health Education Authority (HEA) in association with the UK Ministry of Agriculture, Fisheries and Food (MAFF) and Department of Health (DOH), *Eight Guidelines for a Healthy Diet. A Guide for Nutrition Educators*. HEA in association with MAFF and DOH, 1997, Crown copyright, London.

Chapter 6

1.   Prentice A.M., 'Overeating: The Health Risks'. *Obesity Research*, 9 (4), 2001: 234s–238s.

2.   Rolls, B.J., D. Engell, & L.L. Birch, 'Serving Portion Size Influences 5-year-old But Not 3-year-old Children's Food Intakes'. *Journal of the American Dietetic Association*, 2 (100), 2000: 232–4.

3.   Food Standards Agency and Institute of Food Research, *McCance and Widdowson's The Composition of Foods*. Sixth summary edition. Cambridge: Royal Society of Chemistry, 2002.

Chapter 8
1. British Nutrition Foundation, *Obesity: The Report of the British Nutrition Foundation Task Force.* Blackwell Science, Oxford, 1999.
2. Ibid.
3. Ibid.

Chapter 9
1. Gerrard, D., *Get Up and Go.* Hyndman, Dunedin, 2000.

Chapter 12
1. Stunkard, A.J., & J. Sobal, 'Psychological Consequences'. In K.D. Brownell and C.G. Fairburn, *Eating Disorders and Obesity: A Comprehensive Handbook.* The Guilford Press, New York, 1995.
2. Czajka-Narins, D.M., & E.S. Parham, 'Fear of Fat: Attitudes Toward Obesity'. *Nutrition Today*, January/February 1990: 26–32.
3. Ibid.

INDEX